SOLUTIONS TO CLINICAL MEDICAL CHALLENGES AND PUBLIC HEALTH CHALLENGES

Johnson Mbabazi, MSc FRSPH

and

Mohammad Sattar, General Practitioner MBChB MRCGP

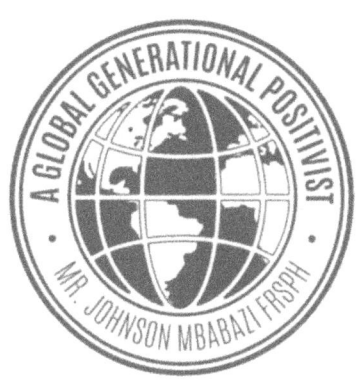

Published by New Generation Publishing in 2021

ISBN: 978-1-80031-077-3

www.newgeneration-publishing.com

New Generation Publishing

CONTENTS

1

EFFICACY OF DIFFERENT TYPES OF METFORMIN MONO- AND COMBINATION DRUG THERAPIES IN CONTROLLING HbA1c LEVELS IN THE TREATMENT OF TYPE 2 DIABETES IN HUMANS COMPARED WITH THE EFFICACY OF EXERCISE ALONE

Johnson Mbabazi

ABSTRACT

Background: Metformin mono- or combination therapies are the most common form of drug therapies used in managing type 2 diabetes. They are usually prescribed after exercise of some sort has been recommended. It is not always clear exactly how much glycaemic control is achieved by using these drugs or exercise.

Objectives: To assess the relative efficacies of Metformin mono- and combination therapies and exercise in controlling diabetes type 2.

Search strategy: Trials were identified by searching Pubmed and conducting manual searches of bibliographies.

Selection Criteria: Randomised controlled trials and retrospective studies investigating the use of Metformin mono- or combination therapies in the treatment of diabetes type 2 with the reduction of HbA1c as a primary outcome.

Data Collection and Analysis: As far as could be obtained, mean changes in HbA1c levels were obtained from all the trials and the percentage of participants who achieved HbA1c levels ≤7% were noted. Any side effects were also recorded.

Main results: Seven trials including six randomised controlled trials and one retrospective study involving a total of 1807 patients. The trials lasted between 14 weeks and 52 weeks. Metformin mono- and combination therapies were shown to achieve mean reductions in HbA1c levels of between 0.6% and 2.7% compared to a mean reduction of 0.6% when using exercise alone.

Conclusion: Exercise constitutes a clinically significant first line treatment of diabetes type 2 especially in its mild forms achieving both noteworthy reductions in HbA1c levels and ameliorating the effects of the disease. The use of Metformin in mono- or combination therapies however causes superior glycaemic control with reduction in mean HbA1c levels of up to 2.7%. This can be particularly useful when treating acute diabetes type 2.

INTRODUCTION

Aim

This review aims to compare the efficacy of treating diabetes type 2 with Metformin as compared to the efficacy of treating it with exercise alone as reported in the existing systematic review by Thomas D., Elliott E. J. and Naughton G. A (2009) in the Cochrane library.

This particular review by Thomas D. et al, on treatment with exercise was selected as it is the only available review that investigates the treatment of diabetes type 2 in adult patients using exercise alone.

Null hypotheses

There will be no significant difference in the efficacy of treating diabetes type 2 with Metformin as compared with the efficacy of exercise alone as reported in the systematic review by Thomas D., Elliott E. J. and Naughton G. A (2009) in the Cochrane Library.

Epidemiology

Approximately 220 million people worldwide suffer from diabetes. Of these, 90% or about 198 million have Diabetes type 2. Unfortunately, the number of patients is on the rise and is expected to reach about 5.6% of the world population by 2030 (WHO, 2010).

In the United Kingdom about 2.3 million adults currently live with diabetes type 2 and an average of 180,000 new cases are diagnosed yearly. This considerable number of new cases is due mainly to increasing obesity and unhealthy lifestyles. Unhealthy lifestyles involve little or no exercise, improper diet and stress.

The likelihood of developing diabetes increases with age and in the UK one in twenty people over 65 and around one in five people over 85 have diabetes (Diabetes UK, 2010). Most of these patients are obese and physically inactive. This observed increase in prevalence with age remained unexplained for a long period. Recent research however, attributes this to increasing mitochondrial damage and a buildup of muscle lipids in the ageing which causes muscle insulin resistance, a major basis of diabetes type 2 (Shulman, G.I. et al, 2010). This damage is due mainly to oxidative stress and reducing mitochondrial oxidative stress would be very important in treating age-related insulin resistance.

Diabetes type 2 is more common in Asians, Africans and Afrocaribbeans with up to 20% of Asians in the UK and 17% of the Afrocaribbean population diagnosed with the disease. People from these ethnic groups are also more likely to develop complications from the disease. This observation has for long been explained by the thrifty gene hypotheses which holds that these ethnic groups inherited certain genes that enable them cope better with cycles of feast and famine but make it harder for them to lose weight. An example of such a gene is the CRTC3 gene which affects obesity (Canettieri, G. et al, 2008). All this exposes an important genetic dimension of the disease.

Statistics from America indicate that 7.8% of the population (23.6 million) there lives with diabetes, with 1.6 million new cases being diagnosed yearly. In the United States, increasing obesity and double digit growth rates in yearly diabetes type 2 diagnoses figures mean burgeoning demands on public health resources. Diabetes type 2 is a leading cause of morbidity and mortality in the USA principally because of its associated renal, neuropathic and heart diseases and in recent years diabetes care has been known to take up one seventh of the US health care budget.

This pressure on public health resources is even more exacting in developing countries where though the prevalence rates are lower than in developed countries, increasing urbanization, adoption of western lifestyles and foods and economic advancements are leading to a projected increase in incidence rates of 170% between 1995 and 2025 (King H. et al, 2008). In 2010, the countries with the highest prevalence in the world are Bahrain, United Arab Emirates, Nauru, Saudi Arabia and Mauritius according to the International Diabetes Federation.

Other factors affecting the prevalence of Type 2 diabetes include environmental factors, Race, Sex and Age. It is more prevalent amongst Asians, Blacks, Native Americans and Hispanic people mostly because of diet types and a higher relative incidence of obesity amongst these groups. Diabetes type 2 is also slightly more prevalent in older women than in age related men because changes in oestrogen and other hormone levels occurring around menopause affect blood sugar levels. It is also more common in people over 40 years old and in much older people is more likely to produce the complications mentioned above because of impaired immune systems.

The preceding statistics are shocking and examining possible solutions to the diabetes epidemic and establishing a single protocol for diabetes management has become an important priority for national and global organisations and diabetes research centres. Several contemporary approaches are used at the moment and include lifestyle changes, exercise, nutrition and pharmacological drugs.

Many organisations and National health bodies worldwide are involved in diabetic research, the most prominent of which are the Center for Disease Control and Prevention, World Health Organisation, International Diabetes Federation, American Diabetes Association, Diabetic Research Institute, Food and Drug Administration and the National Institute for Clinical Excellence. In recent years, research collaboration instead of competition has been stepped up between these associations to develop and realise new concepts in diabetes type 2 control. The IDF for example brings together over 200 national diabetes organisations in 160 countries.

Background

Definition of the condition, causes, long term effects and treatment

Diabetes type 2 is a metabolic disorder caused by a defect in insulin secretion, insulin action or both. Due to this deficiency in insulin performance, Diabetes type 2 is characterised by an increased blood glucose concentration or hyperglycemia and usually results in several long term complications that vary in magnitude depending on the abnormality of the blood sugar levels.

The most common long term complication is damage to the blood vessels which results in an elevated risk of cardiovascular disease. In diabetes, the high quantities of circulating blood sugars result in the excess glucose molecules attaching themselves to proteins and other molecules in the cells and damaging them. This produces persistent inflammation at cellular levels which in turn causes damage to the fine walls of the capillaries obstructing the circulation of blood and nutrients and starving the organs and tissues of oxygen extending this damage. This is mainly how the heart, kidneys, eyes and nerves are affected by diabetes.

Other conditions associated with the disease include eye problems particularly diabetic retinopathy, glaucoma and cataracts, foot ulcerations, diabetic nephropathy (Damage to the kidneys as a result of high blood sugars or hyperglycaemia), diabetic neuropathy (Damage to the nerves as a result of hyperglycaemia), erectile dysfunction (Caused by nerve, blood and muscle damage in the penis) and fungal infections(Caused by bacteria and fungi flourishing on excess glucose).

At present, type 2 diabetes is considered as an inflammatory process caused by cytokines. Cytokines are tiny cell-signaling protein molecules, produced by the glial cells of the nervous system and which are important in intercellular communication. These cytokines are produced by adipocytes. There is a direct link between adipocytes, obesity and diabetes type 2.

In addition, recent studies have found raised macrophage (White blood cells formed from monocytes in tissues) intrusion in white adipose tissue in diabetes type 2 patients. These macrophages sometimes provoke low level chronic inflammation in the tissues of patients and this inflammation contributes to the insulin resistance observed in diabetes type 2 (Weisberg et al, 2003).

In yet more studies, increasing the levels of the fat hormone leptin has been shown to correct plasma glucose and insulin levels in type 2 diabetic patients deficient in this hormone. (Kozlowska et al, 2010). Harnessing the antidiabetic effects of the fat hormone leptin can therefore be important in treating diabetes type 2. The hormone controls the tracer gene IGFBP2 found in the liver. IGFBP2 has been shown to correct high blood sugar and insulin levels independent of weight loss. Human leptin is a protein composed of 167 amino acids which curbs appetite by acting on receptors in the hypothalamus to surpress the effects of the feeding stimulant neuropeptide and by promoting the production of α-MSH which is an appetite suppressant. Leptin is therefore also associated with weight loss and reduction in food intake.

Another approach to treating diabetes type 2 involves using Tumour Necrosis Factor alpha inhibitors to reduce apoptosis of matrix producing cells and promote diabetic healing, particularly in patients suffering from neuropathy or retinopathy. Tumour Necrosis Factor alpha is a cytokine that is associated with immunity, cell destruction, cell repair and inflammation. High levels are associated with diabetes type 2 as a result of overproduction in adipose tissue. Research is being carried out on the effects of varying the levels of TNF-α on type 2 diabetic conditions like retinopathy, neuropathy and nephropathy. Inhibiting the effects of TNF-α has been shown to decrease the retinal microvascular cell loss observed in diabetic retinopathy (Behl, Y. et al, 2008).

Current research on diabetes is spread amongst several approaches and some of the main ones include:

Improving the current methods for monitoring blood glucose levels like pain free glucose tests and continuous monitoring devices. Amira Medical's new AtLast Blood Glucose System, for example, uses a disposable test strip to collect samples from the forearm and thigh without the need for a finger prick. GlucoWatch Biographer extracts fluid through the skin using tiny electrical pulses and sounds an alarm if blood sugar is dangerously low. It can produce 3 hourly measurements and be worn for 12 hours at a stretch.

Gene therapy is another interesting research route. Researchers have for example identified and isolated a gene called SHIP2 that seems to regulate insulin production.

A protein called pigment epithelium-derived factor or PEDF is being shown to prevent the inflammation of blood vessels in the eye and is being investigated as a treatment for diabetic retinopathy (Life Clinic International, 2010).

Long running clinical trials like the SHOW Trial (Study of Health Outcomes of Weight Loss) studied and analysed the effects of weight loss on the health of 3000 overweight(BMI between 25 and 29.9 kg/m^2) and obese(BMI ≥ 30 kg/m^2) patients with type 2 diabetes over a period of 7 years across 15 diabetic research centres in the USA. This is because despite short term benefits of weight loss in managing diabetes some observational studies showed increased complications and mortality with weight loss.

The SHOW trial is now being followed up with the Look AHEAD (Action of Health in Diabetes) trial which will follow 5145 obese patients with diabetes type 2 over 13.5 years. It is investigating the effects of lifestyle changes designed to achieve weight loss and increase physical activity and exercise in overweight and obese adult type 2 diabetes patients.

Exercise too is being used to manage type 2 diabetes. Recent research concentrates on how different types of exercises (aerobic, anaerobic, stretching and vibration) benefit glycaemic control. These include investigations into how exercise manages diabetes by blood sugar reduction, increased metabolism, and reduction in visceral adipose tissue (Mazzone, T. et al, 2006).

Despite all these research into the aforementioned interventions, drug therapies remain by far the most popular method of controlling type 2 diabetes and the common drug therapies are outlined below.

Meglitinides which help boost the pancreas' production of insulin and lower blood sugar levels. They are taken in pill form and act quickly so patients are able to vary meal types, quantity and frequency with less risk of hyperglycaemia. Two types of meglitinides exist: repaglinide and nateglinide. Repaglinide is taken alongside meals to control blood sugar and nateglinide is taken to prevent blood sugar from spiking after meals. They are relatively expensive and are short-acting so they are often administered second line. Examples include drugs like Prandin® and Starlix®. Some common side effects of meglitinides include nausea, vomiting, hypoglycemia or low blood glucose, weight gain, diarrhoea, joint pain, sinus inflammation and bronchitis.

Sulfonylureas function by stimulating insulin secretion in the pancreas and improving body utilisation of insulin. Sulfonylureas also stop the liver from releasing stored glucose into the patient's blood. Together, these actions help sulfonylureas lower blood sugar and have been known to reduce blood sugar levels by up to 20%. They are occasionally used in combination with Metformin, if metformin alone does not yield enough hyperglycaemic control (McCulloch, D.K. et al, 2010). Sometimes they are used initially in patients with heart, kidney or liver disease and those who drink plenty of alcohol. Examples of Sulfonylureas include Diabenese®, Orinase® and Glucotrol®. Some common side effects include sudden hypoglycaemia, weight gain, headaches and abdominal disorders.

Thiazolidinediones function by increasing the sensitivity of the insulin receptor sites in liver cells, muscle and fat and allowing for better absorption of glucose. This improves the patient's sensitivity to insulin. Thiazolidinediones also reduce the liver's production of glucose (McCulloch, D.K et al, 2009). Together these aspects help improve glycaemic control. These drugs are administered orally and are often used second line in combination with other medicines. Some examples include Rosiglitazone(Avandi®) and Pioglitazone(Actos®) and common side effects include anaemia, body pain, pulmonary edema, fatigue, jaundice and weight gain. (American Diabetes Association, 2010)

GLP (Glucagon-like peptide)-agonists are common second line treatments for diabetes mellitus type 2 and are usually administered with other oral medications. GLP agonists function by binding to a membrane GLP receptor and as a consequence of this, insulin release from the pancreatic beta cells is increased. They are commonly used when a patient is not being sufficiently helped by other oral treatments particularly in diaobese patients who are gaining weight on other oral treatments. (NHS Guidelines, 2010) Some examples include Byetta® and Victoza®. Common side effects include nausea, a feeling of fullness, nervousness, decreased appetite and increased sweating.

Alpha-glucosidase inhibitors function by reducing the amount of glucose absorbed in the intestines and this prevents blood sugar levels from spiking after meals. They also help lower blood cholesterol and are taken three times daily alongside meals. Some examples include Precose® and Glyset® and common side effects include diarrhea, flatulence, hypoglycaemia and lightheadedness.

Dipeptidyl peptidase-4 inhibitors (DPP-4) which help the body produce more insulin after meals. They function by raising levels of incretin hormones, which in turn decreases glucagon release and thereby blood sugar levels. Incretin hormones also stimulate insulin production. Some examples include Januvia®, Galvus® and Onglyza® and common side effects are upper respiratory tract infections, urinary tract infections and headaches.

However, Metformin is the main drug. Metformin belongs to the class of Biguanides and is usually the first drug prescribed to newly diagnosed patients because it is relatively less expensive and has the added advantage of not causing hypoglycaemia (NHS Guidelines, 2010).

Metformin functions by improving the body's efficiency in using insulin, reducing gluconeogenesis and decreasing intestinal absorption of glucose. This is achieved by activating the hepatic enzyme AMPK(AMP-Activated Protein Kinase that in vital in insulin signaling and in the metabolism of glucose and lipids. This activation of AMPK results in an increase in SHP (Small heterodimer partner – a nuclear receptor controlling the transfer of genetic information from DNA to mRNA or Messenger Ribonucleic acid). The increase in SHP then inhibits the expression of PEPCK and GLC-6-Pase, which are gluconeogenic genes in the liver. The increase in AMPK also activates GLUT4 or Glucose Transporter type 4 which is a protein found in fatty tissue and skeletal muscle. GLUT4 is vital in controlling how glucose is absorbed into the cell and its increased expression caused by Metformin helps in decreasing the intestinal absorption of insulin in the first instance.

Some metformin drugs include Glucophage®, Gumetza®, Riomet® and Fortamet®. For longer term sufferers who are being treated with insulin, the combination of insulin and metformin results in better blood glucose control (Wulffele, M.G. et al, 2002). Metformin is most often administered to type 2 diabetic patients who are obese and/or are resistant to insulin (Li, D. et al, 2009). Some common side effects of metformin include diarrhea, nausea, abdominal discomfort, indigestion and headaches.

Need for the review

Over the years diabetes type 2 has gradually risen to become a global epidemic. Steadily rising worldwide obesity figures, exceeding 55% in certain countries mean that this type of diabetes which is closely linked to obesity will remain a major concern for the coming decades and that ever more efficient methods must be used to combat it.

The drug therapies mentioned above, namely Meglitinides, Metformin, Sulfonylureas, Insulin, Thiazolidinediones, GLP agonists and Alpha-glucosidase inhibitors are effective and are long established in controlling type 2 diabetes (Wulffele, M.G. et al, 2002). Varying combinations of these drugs have been shown to improve glycaemic control in numerous clinical trials. In one case, a combination therapy of Metformin and Insulin was shown to improve glycaemic control while reducing insulin requirements and weight gain (Wulffele, M.G. et al, 2002). Metformin and some Meglitinides have also been shown to demonstrably reduce HbA1c by 0.5% and over. A reduction of HbA1c of about 1% results in a 21% reduction of diabetes related complications or deaths (Black C. et al, 2009).

However, Conventional pharmacological drug therapies exist for diabetes type 2 but all drugs taken long term cause problems and side effects therefore exploring non drug ways, like exercise, of managing non-insulin dependent diabetes mellitus would be beneficial. Additionally, exploding costs of drug therapies mean that alternative therapies and combination therapies must be examined to reduce the burden of diabetes type 2 on national health resources.

Exercise, alongside lifestyle (diet) changes, represents the first line of support against Diabetes type 2 (NHS Guidelines, 2010). NHS guidelines recommend the use of exercise in managing diabetes prevention and cure before proceeding to drug therapies. Exercise reduces weight and blood glucose and fatty acids are burned. Diabetes is more common in people who are overweight ($25 \text{ kg/m}^2 < \text{BMI} \leq 29.9 \text{ kg/m}^2$) and obese ($\text{BMI} \geq 30 \text{ kg/m}^2$) than in those who are not. Normal BMI is ≤ 25 kg/m^2. Some research studies have found up to 90% of those who are newly diagnosed with type 2 diabetes to be over their ideal weight as indicated by BMI. According to Frank B et al, 2001 being overweight or obese was found to be the most important single predictor for developing diabetes. Diet restrictions and the accompanying weight loss are therefore an important first step in managing the disease.

Exercise has also long been used as a therapeutic intervention for the prevention and treatment of insulin resistance or impaired glucose tolerance connected with Type 2 diabetes. It has been shown to increase insulin sensitivity by up to 30% (Hawley 2004). According to McCulloch, D.K. et al, (2005), even regular exercise without weight loss has been shown to substantially reduce visceral fat and Type 2 diabetic symptoms.

Diabetic control

Control of diabetes type 2 is best assessed by using an HbA1c test. Glucose combines with Haemoglobin in red blood cells to produce a molecule called HbA1c and measuring the level of HbA1c can give a good indication of the average level of plasma glucose over 8 to 12 weeks which is the average life span of red blood cells. Normal non-diabetic levels lie between 3.5% and 5.5% with levels of 6.5% considered good for diabetic patients (NHS Guidelines, 2010).

METHODOLOGY

This systematic review alongside other systematic reviews will identify as much as possible of the existing published research studies relevant to the particular research question and by deploying explicit and systematic methods establish what can be deduced from these studies. This will be accomplished in a series of steps which include specifying the objectives before hand and selecting the criteria for including studies. That will then be followed by a detailed and systematic search for studies using a series of reproducible steps and an assessment of the studies included. The finding shall then be compared and presented in an orderly manner relative to the initial objectives.

The literature review method employed here has the distinct advantage of requiring only very few resources. There is however a risk of bias due to selective availability of data.

A Cochrane search was carried out and there was no existing systematic review on this topic. The search revealed no presented reviews.

To get relevant information on primary articles and clinical trials used in this systematic review, an electronic literature search was carried out. It used the Pubmed database purposeful on obtaining primary articles. The search terms used included Type 2 diabetes, Metformin (Biguanides), glycaemic control (HbA1c) or glycosylated Hb levels.

To identify existing randomised controlled trials using Metformin to control diabetes type 2.

To establish the number of patients and their types (diaobese, gender, adult, infants, pregnant etc.)

To deduce if Metformin or exercise is efficient in treating and managing type 2 diabetes by directly comparing HbA1c values.

The efficacy of different types of diabetes treatments can be compared using numerous variables. Several researchers have used HbA1c, FPG (Fasting Plasma Glucose), BMI (Body Mass Index), changes from baseline in lipoproteins and triglycerides, changes from baseline in systolic and diastolic pressures and many others.

This review will directly compare the efficacies of Metformin and exercise using the HbA1c test only which gives a measure of glycosulated haemoglobin.

Table 1. Search strategy 1

Inclusion criteria	Justification
The articles that had to be human based studies.	It would be inadequate to compare efficacy based on glycaemic control in animals to glycaemic control achieved by exercise in humans.
In studies the participants had to be over 18.	This was to exclude children and facilitate a like for like comparison with the adult participants in the exercise review. Also Type 1 diabetes is more common in children.
Variations in BMI from 20 kg/m^2 to 40 kg/m^2.	To exclude patients that were underweight. Underweight ≤18.5 kg/m^2; Normal weight = 18.5–24.9 kg/m^2; Overweight = 25–29.9 kg/m^2; Obesity ≥30 kg/m^2.
Studies involving any combination drug therapies including Metformin. Trials had to include Metformin at least even if they were combination drug therapies.	This was to be as inclusive as possible and involve more participants.
Studies in which participants had been diagnosed with diabetes for at least 3 months but no longer than 10 years.	Patients have been observed to develop resistance to single agent therapies over time.
Studies involving participants with other major underlying health conditions or those taking long term medications	To exclude any possible interference in establishing the efficacy contributions of Metformin.
Articles that had to include the search terms in the Title or Abstract.	Articles had to be mainly about Metformin as a main drug.
Primary articles (Had to be Randomised control trials or retrospective studies).	Access to original data was important so review studies were excluded.
All articles had to be published later than the year 1995.	To ensure that the research was current.
All articles had to be written in English only.	No access to translation facilities.
Trials had to be fully published.	To eliminate extra costs in purchasing journals.

It was important to exclude any review studies, in order to include as much original primary data as possible in this systematic review. This systematic review was supposed to be the first review of its type.

Using these inclusion and exclusion criteria, an initial electronic search (using Pubmed database in this case) revealed the following number of articles possibly relevant to this review study. This is shown in Table 2 below.

Table 2. Search strategy 2

Search term	Number of hits
Type 2 diabetes	1170
Metformin (Biguanides)	257
HbA1c (Glycaemic Control)	487
Type 2 Diabetes AND Metformin	151 (152 minus one review)
Type 2 Diabetes AND HbA1c	331
Type 2 Diabetes, Metfomin AND HbA1c	69

The 69 articles obtained in this initial search were then hand searched and narrowed down further considering relevance and using the following quality assessment measures. The studies had to be longer term studies of over 12 weeks. 12 weeks is the average lifespan of red blood cells and measuring HbA1c levels over periods shorter than this gives only an incomplete picture of the overall changes in glycosulated haemoglobin levels. The studies had to include at least 70 patients. This was considered to be a reasonable minimum sample size necessary to add both credibility and generalisability to the results. The studies also had to compare the efficacy of Metformin (Monotherapy or Combined therapy) directly to placebo using HbA1c results. Measuring HbA1c is the most common way of diagnosing and measuring type 2 diabetes, giving an indication of how advanced the diabetes is in a given patient. The results sections were particularly important and the articles had to have detailed results, preferably in graph or table format. The quality of the references were also taken into account.

This manual search result in the 7 articles listed in the Table 3 below.

Search carried out on 1/03/2019.

DISCUSSION

Garber, A.J. et al, 2003

This trial examined patients with type 2 diabetes who had inadequate glycemic control of glycosylated hemoglobin (HbA1C) of between 7% and 12% with diet and exercise alone. It compared the efficacies of treatment with glyburide/metformin tablets versus metformin therapy or glyburide monotherapy. 486 patients were randomised to receive glyburide/metformin tablets (1.25/250 mg), metformin (500 mg), or glyburide (2.5 mg). Changes in A1C were measured after 16 weeks.

Glyburide/metformin tablets caused a mean reduction in A1C from baseline (−2.27%) versus Metformin monotherapy (−1.53%) and glyburide (−1.90%) monotherapy (P = 0.0003). First-line treatment with Metformin therefore resulted in clinically significant glycaemic control which could be further enhanced by administering metformin in a combination therapy as glyburide/metformin tablets.

This trial is very well done in that the patients were all classified beforehand into gender, age and BMI. Also a record was made of how long beforehand each patient had been diagnosed and what levels of glycaemic control had previously been achieved with exercise and diet alone excluding drug therapy. The trial also included a large sample size and was of an adequate duration of 16 weeks to permit proper conclusions on changes in glycaemic control to be reached.

Possible weaknesses in the trial stem mostly from its reliance on patient input. Patient diagnosis history (length of illness) was obtained directly from patient and the HbA1c measurements were made by the patients themselves leading to possible inaccuracies. Also the calculation of the mean daily glucose levels using 4 fingerstick measurements taken independently before breakfast, lunch, supper and at bedtime could have led to patients misrepresenting measurements making the results less reliable.

Chiasson, J.L. et al, 2001

This multicentre, double-blind, placebo controlled study investigates the efficacy of metformin in combination with miglitol in improving glycaemic control in outpatients in whom type 2 diabetes had not been adequately controlled by diet alone in Canadian test centres. 324 patients were randomised, after 8 weeks of a placebo run-in period, to treatment with either metformin alone, miglitol alone,

Table 3. Extractions Table - Shows results of the seven articles critically evaluated

Title of Journal Article and Authors	Study Design/ Methods	Participants	Study Details	Results
Efficacy of Glyburide/ Metformin Tablets Compared with Initial Monotherapy in Type 2 Diabetes. **Garber, A.J. et al, 2003**	Multicentre, Double-blinded trial.	Investigated 486 patients with high HbA1c levels of greater than 7% but less than 12%. It included 213 men and 273 women. Patients had to be between 20 and 78, have had a diagnosis of diabetes for at least 3 months	Patients were randomised to receive 500 mg of Metformin, a combination of glyburide and Metformin (1.25 mg/250 mg) or glyburide only (1.25 mg) over 16 weeks.	Glyburide/Metformin caused the greatest mean reduction in A1C from baseline (−2.27%) versus metformin (−1.53%) and glyburide (−1.90%) monotherapy
The Synergistic Effect of Miglitol Plus Metformin Combination Therapy in the Treatment of Type 2 Diabetes. **Chiasson, J.L. et al, 2001**	Multicentre, Randomised, Double-blind placebo controlled study.	318 patients. HbA1c was greater than or equal to 7.2% but less than or equal to 9.5%. The patients included 240 men and 84 women. The patients ages ranged from 47 to 67	Randomised 83 to placebo, 83 to Metformin, 82 to Miglitol and 76 to Metformin and Miglitol over 36 weeks. A clinically significant response in this trial was taken by the authors to be either a greater than or equal to 15% reduction in baseline HbA1c or an HbA1c level of less than 7%.	The final mean ± Stand Error of Mean for HbA1c values was 7.3±0.1% for Metformin, 8.2±0.2%, 6.9±0.1% for a combination of metformin and miglitol and 8.5±0.1% for placebo.
Triple Therapy in Type 2 Diabetes. Insulin glargine or rosiglitazone added to combination therapy of sulfonylurea plus metformin in insulin naive patients. **Rosenstock, J. et al, 2006.**	Randomised, open-label trial	Involved 216 participants. These included 112 men and 104 women. The subjects ages ranged from 40 to 65.	Metformin in combination with sulfonylurea and one other add- on drug(Rosiglitazone or Insuline glargine) was compared across 42 US centres.	HbA1c level improvements were comparable in both groups. 49% of patients in the Metformin Sulfonylurea Rosiglitazone combined therapy achieved ADA recommended levels of ≤7%.
Efficacy of Metformin in patients with non-insulin dependent diabetes mellitus. **Defronzo, R.A. et al, 1995**	Randomised, double-blind, controlled study. Protocol comparing Metformin to placebo in 289 type 2 diabetes patients.	Involved 289 type 2 diabetes patients. They comprised 124 males and 168 females. The mean age of the participants was 53.1 years.	Metformin(n=143) at a maximum daily of 2250 mg or placebo(n=146) over 29 weeks.	After 29 weeks, 143 patients on Metformin showed HbA1c values of 7.1± 0.1% versus values of 8.6 ±0.2% for 146 patients on placebo. The values for Metformin approach those recommended by the ADA for drug therapies.

14

Title & Author	Study Design	Participants	Methodology	Results
Twelve and 52 week Efficacy of the Dipeptidyl Peptidase IV Inhibitor LAF237 IN Metformin-Treated Patients with type 2 diabetes **Ahren, B. et al, 2004**	Randomised, Double blind, placebo controlled trial.	107 type 2 diabetes The patients ages ranged from 42 to 67 and they were divided into 73 males and 34 females.	51 Patients were given a combination of placebo and Metformin at 1500–3000 once daily. 56 Patients were given a combination of LAF237 and Metformin at a similar dose. The patients started out with HbA1c levels of >7% but ≤9.5%. Patients were investigated over up to 12 weeks and then 72 of them for a further 40 weeks.	The combination of Metformin and LAF237 resulted in the best glycaemic control. 41.7% of patients taking LAF237 and Metformin attained HbA1c levels of <7% compared to only 10.7% for those on Metformin and placebo.
Improvements in Glycemic Control in Type 2 Diabetes Patients Switched From Sulfonylurea Coadministered With Metformin to Glyburide-Metformin Tablets **Duckworth, W. et al, 2003**	Randomised, Multicentre, cohort study examining the efficacy of Metformin amongst servicemen and veterans.	This paper examined 72 patient records. The patients were divided into 70 males and 2 females. The mean age was 62 years. Patient records went back 16 weeks.	Compared the efficacy of glyburide-metformin tablets to non-tablet therapies of both Metformin plus glyburide and Metformin plus Glipizide. The glyburide-metformin tablets were administered at a dose of 20 mg/2000 mg and in the non-tablet form, the maximum daily dose of Glyburide was 20 mg, 40 mg for Glipizide and 2000 mg for Metformin.	Metformin in combination with Glyburide resulted in an improved mean reduction in HbA1c of 0.6% from a mean baseline of 7.9% (±SD 1.7).
Treatment With the Human Once-Weekly Glucagon-Like Peptide-1 Analog Taspoglutide in Combination With Metformin Improves Glycemic Control and Lowers Body Weight in Patients With Type 2 Diabetes Inadequately Controlled With Metformin Alone. **Nauck, A.M. et al, 2009**	Double-blind placebo-controlled study.	297 patients were involved. The patients ranged in age from 42 to 64 years. Involved 154 females and 143 males.	It investigated possible improvements in glycaemic control for patients inadequately helped by Metformin alone - by combining their Metformin treatment with Taspoglutide at varying doses. Glycaemic control was measured for 297 patients on 1500 mg daily dose of Metformin and varying subcutaneous doses of taspoglutide against placebo. Trial lasted 14 weeks.	All patients who received Taspoglutide recorded statistically significant improvements in glycaemic control. 44% of all those on the taspoglutide achieved ADA recommended HbA1c levels of <7%. Patients with higher starting HbA1c levels of ≥8% recorded the largest improvements.

miglitol in addition to metformin or placebo for a total of 36 weeks. The miglitol was administered at 100 mg and metformin at 500 mg three times a day. The main criterion used in measuring efficacy was a change in HbA1c from baseline to the end of treatment.

The highest reduction in mean placebo subtracted HbA1c was 21.78% and occurred with the combination of miglitol and metformin followed by 21.25% for metformin alone.

This experiment was particularly detailed in recording diagnosis history, age, weight, gender, ethnicity, BMI and previous drug therapy use.

Possible weaknesses include the fact that several patients were long term diabetics of over 14 years and that the sample size was predominantly Caucasian.

Rosenstock, J. et al, 2006

This study examined 216 type 2 diabetes patients across 42 US test centres. It examined the efficacy of a combined therapy of Sulfonylurea Metformin and Rosiglitazone to a combined therapy of Sulfonylurea Metmormin and Insulin Glargine in diabetes type 2 patients who had never previously been treated with insulin.

Metformin was administered at a constant dose of 2000 mg/day. A daily dose of a Sulfonylurea at ≤50% of the recommended daily dose was also kept constant. An initial daily oral dose of Rosiglitazone at 4 mg/day which was gradually increased to an average of 7.1±1.7 mg/day was administered to the first group of 112 patients. Insulin glargine was titrated at an initial nightly (Bedtime 2100–2300) dose of 10 IU/day which was increased to 38.5±26.5 IU/day at the end of the experiment for the second group of 104 patients.

Both triple combined therapies produced comparable results with 49% of patients in the Metformin Sulfonylurea Rosiglitazone combined therapy achieving ADA recommended levels of ≤7% compared to 48% for Metformin Insuline Glargine patients.

Examining the paper revealed certain weaknesses. The ethnicity of the patients was not recorded giving no insight into variations in incidence, efficacy and side effects for the different races.

As a strength, the paper gives detailed information about the cost of the different therapies at varying doses.

Defronzo, R.A. et al, 1995

This randomised controlled trial examined 289 diabetes type 2 patients who did not achieve adequate glycaemic control with diet restrictions. They were randomised into two groups of 143 to receive Metformin at a maximum daily dose of 2250 mg and 146 to receive placebo over 29 weeks. The patients were classed as moderately obese with the BMI ranging from 28.9 kg/m^2 to 30.2 kg/m^2. The mean age was 53.1 years

After 29 weeks, 143 patients on Metformin showed HbA1c values of 7.1± 0.1% versus values of 8.6 ±.0.2% for 146 patients on placebo. The values for Metformin approach those recommended by the ADA for drug therapies.

31 patients in the Metformin group and 41 patients in the placebo group recorded adverse effects. These effects included diarrhoea and nausea and were only characterised as severe in <8% of those on Metformin and <4% of those on placebo.

Strong points of this trial include the detailed statistical analysis of all the variables like age, BMI and HbA1c levels and that it details the adverse effects and the number of patients in each group who suffered from them in the course of the trial.

Several weaknesses were observed however. These include no reference to ethnicity giving no insight into incidence and variations along ethnic lines. Also there are no restrictions on the upper limit of HbA1c levels at the outset of the experiment. The patients do not appear to have been classified into groups according to their initial HbA1c levels so it is impossible to deduce and compare how much glycaemic control is achieved for each treatment group.

Ahren, B. et al, 2004

In this randomised placebo controlled trial the 12 and 52 week efficacies of 2 combination therapies were investigated. The first included a combination of Metformin at a daily dose of 1500–3000 mg and LAF237 (Dipeptidyl Peptidase IV Inhibitor). The second included a combination of Metformin at an identical dose and a placebo. 107 (56 on Metformin/LAF237 and 51 on Metformin/placebo) patients took part in the first 12 weeks after which 71 patients(42 on Metformin/LAF237 and 29 on Metformin/placebo) agreed to extend the study for another 40 weeks.

The combination of Metformin and LAF237 resulted in better glycaemic control. At the end of the experiment, 41.7% of patients taking LAF237 and Metformin had HbA1c levels of <7% compared to only 10.7% for those on Metformin and placebo.

Changes in baseline HbA1c of -0.6±0.1% were observed in the group randomised to LAF237 with an average baseline level of 7.7±0.1%. No changes in baseline were observed for the group on placebo with baseline averaging at 7.9±0.1%.

This paper was particularly strong in that it included a relatively detailed safety and tolerability map for both therapies. For example, 2 patients on Metformin and LAF237 suffered one episode of hypoglycemia each during the first 12 weeks compared to none for Metformin plus placebo.

As a weakness there was no classification with regards to ethnicity giving no insight into incidence and variations along ethnic lines.

Duckworth, W. et al, 2003

In this retrospective study, the patient records of 72 veterans and servicemen across 4 medical centres in the US were examined. The main purpose was to establish any efficacy improvements from switching patients on Metformin administered in combination with a Sulfonylurea (Glyburide and Glipizide) in non-tablet form to Metformin-Glyburide tablets.

The maximum daily dose before the switch was less than 2000 mg for Metformin, 40 mg for Glipizide and 20 mg for Glypuride. The dose of Glyburide to Metformin in the tablets was 20 mg to 2000 mg respectively.

The participants had a mean age of 62 years and a mean BMI of 32.9 kg/m^2. They were predominantly male and white: 70 males and 2 females with 52 recorded as white, 8 as african American, 3 as Hispanic and 9 as other.

After a mean follow up period of 196 days, Metformin-Glyburide tablets resulted in an improved mean reduction in HbA1 c of 0.6% from a mean baseline of 7.9% (±SD 1.7). 6 patients suffered from complications on the non-tablet therapies and 11 suffered complications after the switch to glyburide-metformin tablets.

One major strength in this study is the depth of the statistical analysis. For example, all variables in the study like age, BMI and doses are examined closely and expressed as mean values.

Some weaknesses are immediately apparent in this study however: the sample size of 72 patients is small therefore it is hard to generalise results. Also because all the patients were either servicemen or veterans, the results might not be immediately transferable to the general population. The retrospective nature of the study also means a great deal of data was not collected and no controls could be enforced. For example, it was not possible to ensure and average daily dose of the combination therapies prior to the switch to Glyburide-metformin tablets.

Nauck, A.M. et al, 2009

297 type 2 diabetes patients not obtaining sufficient glycaemic control from a daily dose of Metformin at 1500 mg were randomized to receive 8 weeks of treatment with Taspoglutide at varying doses and intervals in combination with their metformin dose.

148 patients were randomised to receive weekly subcutaneous injections of placebo or taspoglutide at 5 mg, 10 mg or 20 mg. The remaining 149 patients were randomised to receive taspoglutide at doses of 5 mg, 10 mg or 20 mg once every 2 weeks.

The patients had starting values of HbA1c of >7% and ≤9.5% and all patients who received Taspoglutide recorded statistically significant improvements in glycaemic control. 44% of all those on the taspoglutide achieved ADA recommended HbA1c levels of <7%. Patients with higher starting HbA1c levels of ≥8% recorded the largest improvements.

One strong point about this study is that it details all the side effects and adverse effects that were incurred by patients during the study and the number of patients in each treatment regimen who suffered from them. Examples of adverse effects included nausea, vomiting, decreased appetite, headaches, diarrhea, dyspepsia (impaired digestion) and abdominal distension.

Some of the weaknesses that stand out include; the 8 week treatment period is clinically insufficient to determine the complete glycaemic control benefits of using the Metformin-Taspoglutide combination therapy. This is because 8 weeks are much less than the 12 week life span of erythrocytes red blood cells. Also there is no mention of ethnicity so no insight into incidence and variations along ethnic lines can be drawn. Additionally, the unknown ratio of the sexes amongst the final 297 participants who were randomised into the various treatment groups also limits insight into incidence and variations between the sexes.

Thomas D. et al, 2009

These researchers investigated the clinical benefits of exercise against no exercise at all in managing diabetes type 2. The resulting systematic review included 14 trials and 377 patients and looked at different protocols lasting between 2 and 12 months.

The types of exercise included in this study were aerobic exercise, general fitness exercise and resistance building exercise. A close look at all 14 protocols revealed that reductions in HbA1c levels of up to 0.6% could be achieved with exercise alone even without accompanying weight loss. This difference is both of clinical and statistical significance.

Upon examining subgroups, HbA1c reductions were greater in shorter term studies than in long term studies with reductions of up to 0.8% for trials shorter than 12 weeks and 0.7% for trials shorter than 16 weeks. It could also be shown that upon follow-up after up to one year, this improved levels of HbA1c were maintained (Yeater, 1990).

Also no adverse effects were recorded across all 14 protocols examined with only 2 of them referring to initial muscle soreness as a major complaint (Baldi 2003 and Dunstan 2002). Lack of time was another complaint experienced (Loimaala, 2003).

Table 4. Comparison - Exercise versus no exercise, Outcome Glycated haemoglobin (%).

Analysis : Comparison 1 Exercise versus no exercise, Outcome Glycated haemoglobin (%).

Review: Exercise for type 2 diabetes mellitus

Comparison: 1 Exercise versus no exercise

Outcome: Glycated haemoglobin (%)

Study or Subgroup	Exercise N	Mean(SD)	Control N	Mean(SD)	Weight	Mean Difference IV, Fixed, 95% CI
Wing 1988b	13	8.2(1.08)	15	9(1.16)	12.0%	-0.80 [-1.63, 0.03]
Baldi 2003	9	8.4(1.8)	9	8.4(8)	3.0%	0.0 [-1.66, 1.66]
Cuff 2003	10	6.8(1.26)	9	6.87(1.2)	6.7%	-0.07 [-1.18, 1.04]
Dela 2004	9	8.2(1.8)	7	8.5(1.59)	3.0%	-0.3 [-1.96, 1.36]
Dunstan 1998	11	8(1.66)	10	8.3(2.21)	2.9%	-0.3 [-1.98, 1.38]
Dunstan 2002	16	6.9(1)	13	7.1(1.1)	13.8%	-0.2 [-0.97, 0.57]
Loimaala 2003	24	7.6(1.4)	25	8.3(1.4)	13.4%	-0.7 [-1.48, 0.08]
Maiorana 2002	16	7.9(1.2)	16	8.5(1.6)	8.6%	-0.6 [-1.58, 0.38]
Mourier 1997	10	6.2(0.63)	11	7.7(1.33)	10.7%	-1.5 [-2.38, -0.62]
Raz 1994	19	11.7(2.6)	19	12.9(4.2)	1.7%	-1.2 [-3.42, 1.02]
Ronnemaa 1986	13	8.6(1.9)	12	9.9(1.7)	4.1%	-1.3 [- 2.71, 0.11]
Tessier 2000	19	7.6(1.2)	20	7.8(1.5)	11.4%	-0.2 [-1.05, 0.65]
Tsujiuchi 2002	16	7.33(1.09)	10	8.17(1.3)	8.8%	-0.84 [-1.81, 0.13]
Total (95% CI)	**185**		**176**		**100%**	**-1.3 [- 2.71, 0.11]**

Heterogeneity: Chi2 = 9.27, df = 12 (P = 0.68); I2 =0.0%

Test for overall effect: Z = 4.25 (P = 0.000022)

Thomas D. et al, 2009

The Table 4 above details the differences in HbA1c levels from 13 of the 14 protocols used in the systematic review by Thomas D. et al, 2009. Despite the relatively small sample sizes of each experiment, across all experiments a definite and significant glycaemic control benefit can be immediately observed. The review of exercise in treating diabetes type 2 by Thomas D, et al, 2009 showed a reduction in glycated haemoglobin levels of 0.6% HbA1c while as drug trials here have indicated a reduction in HbA1c levels between 0.6% up to 2.7%. Additional benefits of exercise included reduced visceral and subcutaneous adipose tissue, lowered plasma triglycerides and improved insulin response.

RESULTS COMPARISON

A close look at the systematic review by Thomas D. reveals a mean improvement in glycaemic control across 13 of the exercise trials of –0.62%. This is shown in Table 4. Though in most cases the ADA recommended level of 7% was not attained with exercise alone, a reduction of this magnitude is of major clinical importance. Further examination also exposes other important benefits of exercise outlined above including most importantly the near absence of side effects.

Garber, A.J. et al, 2003 demonstrated mean reductions in HbA1c of up to 2.7% with glyburide/ metformin tablets, 1.53% with titrated metformin in a monotherapy and up to 1.90% with Glyburide alone. With 62% of patients in the trial on metformin monotherapy achieving recommended HbA1c levels of 7%, this represents a massive improvement when compared to managing type 2 diabetes with exercise alone. This improvement though was accompanied by adverse effects including diarrhoea, abdominal pain, nausea, headaches and upper respiratory infections.

Chiasson, J.L. et al, 2001 achieved mean reductions of HbA1c approaching 1.78% with a combination therapy of metformin and miglitol. In their clinical trial involving 318 patients, mean HbA1c levels at the end of the trials were 8.2 ± 0.2% for Miglitol, 7.3 ± 0.1% for Metformin alone and 6.9 ± 0.1% for Metformin plus Miglitol. This constitutes yet again a considerable improvement in glycaemic control when compared to the mean reduction value of 0.62% for exercise alone. However the patients suffered several adverse effects which included dyspepsia, constipation, abdominal cramps, hypoglycaemia and nausea.

Rosenstock, J. et al, 2006 showed that a combination therapy of Metformin, sulfonylurea and insulin glargine could reduce HbA1c levels by up to 1.7% in insulin naïve patients. Once again this trial revealed the comparative dominance in reducing HbA1c levels with a Metformin combination therapy. 49% of 112 patients on Metformin/Sulfonylurea/Rosiglitazone achieved HbA1c levels of ≤7% and 48% of 104 patients on Metformin/Sulfonylurea/insulin glargine reached HbA1c levels of ≤ 7%. These drug therapies were however came with the following adverse effects: nausea, oedema, weight gain and hypoglycaemia. Over 24 weeks, the cost per patient treated using Metformin/Sulfonylurea/ Rosiglitazone was $1603. This compared with the $1368 it required to treat a patient with Metformin/ Sulfonylurea /insulin glargine. This reveals an advantage of exercise in that is relatively cheaper if the patients went to a gym and can even be free depending on the exercise type.

Defronzo, R. A et al, 1995 demonstrated improvements in HbA1c levels of -1.4 ± 0.1% with a Metformin therapy. After 29 weeks of treatment with metformin143 patients showed a mean HbA1c value of 7.1 ± 0.1% compared to 8.6 ± 0.2% for placebo. This signifies well over twice the average improvement of 0.62% attained by using exercise alone. Several adverse effects like nausea and diarrhoea were experienced by up to 31 of the 143 patients on the metformin therapy.

Ahren, B. et al, 2004 showed the improved benefits of adding the dipeptidyl peptidase IV inhibitor LAF237 to an ongoing Metformin drug treatment. Examining changes in baseline HbA1c levels among patients for up to 12 weeks, they showed that mean improvements of up to 0.6± 0.1% in HbA1c could be achieved with a combination therapy of Metformin and LAF237 with up to 41.7% of the patients on this therapy achieving HbA1c levels of ≤7%. This is comparable to the changes observed with HbA1c but came with the following side effects: cough, urinary tract infection, gastroenteritis, Nasopharyngitis (Inflammation of the nasopharynx) and hypertension.

Duckworth, W. et al, 2003, by examining patient records, showed that improvements in HbA1c levels of between 1.2% and 1.4% could be achieved with a combination therapy of Glyburide-Metformin tablets in patients with acute diabetes type 2 showing HbA1c levels ≥8%. This is a considerable improvement when compared to treating diabetes type 2 with exercise alone which showed an average improvement in HbA1c levels of only 0.62% as shown by Thomas D. et al, 2009. Adverse effects including hypoglycaemia and diabetic foot disease were experienced by some patients using this therapy.

Nauck, A.M. et al, 2009 demonstrated the improvements in glycaemic control that could be achieved by using Metformin in a combination therapy with Taspoglutide. Changes in HbA1c levels of up to 1.2% were observed with this combination therapy with 44% of those on the Metformin-taspoglutide therapy achieving the ADA recommended treatment levels of ≤7%. This is therefore about twice as effective as treating diabetes type 2 with exercise alone as shown by Thomas D. et al, 2009. This therapy though was connected with certain effects for some patients including nausea, vomiting, diarrhoea, dyspepsia, abdominal distension and headaches.

CONCLUSION

Implications for practice

This review concludes that Metformin monotherapy or a combination drug therapy including Metformin is very efficient in managing diabetes type 2. From current research it has been shown that these therapies can significantly reduce glycated haemoglobin levels in the range of between 0.6% and 2.7%. This is of great clinical significance particularly for patients suffering from acute diabetes with HbA1c levels ≥8%. In some patients however these improvements are sometimes accompanied by adverse effects to the alimentary tract causing nausea, vomiting, decreased appetite, headaches, diarrhea, dyspepsia (impaired digestion) and abdominal distension. The trials included in this review used different types of Metformin drug therapies in varying combinations, doses and forms (Titrated, tablets etc.). The most suitable one can therefore be chosen for a patient depending on lifestyle preference, cost and severity of the disease.

From the stand of current research, exercise has been shown to reduce HbA1c levels by up to 0.6%. This is of substantial clinical significance, especially in patients with mild diabetes, where exercise alone would be sufficient in managing the disease and avoiding the need for a drug intervention. For a patient with severe diabetes with an HbA1c value of say 8%, an improvement of 0.6% represents a 60% improvement towards the ADA recommended treatment target for drug therapies of 7%. Additional benefits of treating diabetes with exercise ascertained from current research include the lower cost, fewer side effects, improved insulin sensitivity and reduced visceral and subcutaneous adipose tissue.

Early diagnosis and exercise as a first line treatment would represent an ideal way to manage mild diabetes type 2 and ameliorate the effects of the disease. In later more severe stages, a drug therapy comprising Metformin can then be used to control diabetes type 2. From the stand point of glycaemic control alone drug therapies are more effective than exercise therapy in managing diabetes type 2.

Implications for research

From current research, there is substantial evidence that enhancements in HbA1c control can be achieved long term with both exercise and Metformin mono- and combination therapies.

Almost all studies investigating the benefits of exercise in treating diabetes type 2 have used relatively small sample sizes and had short follow up periods. There is therefore a need to carry out studies involving more participants with post intervention follow ups building up to between 52 weeks and 3 years. This would determine what kind of exercise is most beneficial, if and what kind of exercise can be maintained regularly over long periods, and give detailed insight into changes in attitude towards diabetes and changes to quality of life.

There is a need to research how the side effects of the Metformin therapies can be reduced and even further, a need to detect and investigate possible long term complications of treating type 2 diabetes with Metformin.

With the increasing incidence of type 2 diabetes in children, studies investigating the efficacies of these interventions in children also need to be carried out.

REFERENCES

Ahren, B., Mills, D., Gomis, R., Standl, E., and Schweizer, A. (2004). Twelve- and 52-Week Efficacy of the Dipeptidyl Peptidase IV Inhibitor LAF237 in Metformin-Treated Patients With Type 2 Diabetes. Journal of Diabetes Care. 27 (12), p2874–2879.

Anderson, J.W., Kendall, C.W.C. and Jenkins, D.J.A.. (2003). Importance of Weight Management in Type 2 Diabetes: Review with Meta-analysis of Clinical Studies. Journal of the American College of Nutrition. 22 (5), p331–339.

Baum, K., Votteler, T., and Schiab, J.. (2007). Efficiency of vibration exercise for glycemic control in type 2 diabetes patients. International Journal of Medical Sciences. 3 (4), p159–163.

Behl, Y., Krothapalli, P., Desta, T., DiPiazza, A., Roy, S., and Graves, D.T.. (2008). Diabetes-Enhanced Tumor Necrosis Factor-α Production Promotes Apoptosis and the Loss of Retinal Microvascular Cells in Type 1 and Type 2 Models of Diabetic Retinopathy. The American Journal of Pathology. 172 (5), p1411–1418.

Black, P., McIntyre, L., Royle, P., Shepherd, J., and Thomas, S. (2009). "Meglitide analogues for type 2 diabetes mellitus (Review)." THE COCHRANE COLLABORATON.

Canettieria, G., Coni, S., Guardia, M.D., Nocerino, V., Antonucci, L., Magno, L., Screaton, R., Screpanti, I., Giannini, G., and Gulino, A.. (2009). The coactivator CRTC1 promotes cell proliferation and transformation via AP-1. Journal of cell Biology. 106 (5), p1445–1450.

Chiasson, J.L., Naditch, L., and The Miglitol Canadian University. (2001). The Synergistic Effect of Effect of Miglitol Plus Metformin Combination Therapy in the Treatment of Type 2 Diabetes. The journal of Diabetes Care. 24 (6), p989–994.

Defronzo, R.A. Goodman, A, M., and The Multicentre Metformin Group. (1995). Efficacy of metformin in patients with niddm. The New England Journal of Medicine. 333 (9), p541–549.

Garber, J., Donovan, S., Dandona, P., Bruce, S., and Park, J. (2003). Efficacy of Glyburide/Metformin Tablets Compared with Initial Monotherapy in Type 2 Diabetes. The Journal of Clinical Endocrinology and Metabolism. 88 (8), p3598–3604.

Gottschalk, M., Danne, T., Vlajnic, A., and Cara, J.F. (2007). Glimepiride Versus Metformin as Monotherapy in Pediatric Patients With Type 2 Diabetes. Journal of Diabetes Care. 30 (4), p790–794.

Hawley, J. A. (2004). "Exercise as a therapeutic intervention for the prevention and treatment of insulin resistance." Diabetes/Metabolism Research And Reviews 20: 383–393.

Hills, A.P., Shultz, S.P., Soares, M.J., Byrne, N.M., Hunter, G.R., King, N.A., and Misra, A.. (2009). Obesity Management. Resistance training for obese, type 2 diabetic adults: a review of the evidence.. Obesity reviews. 10 (1), p1–10.

King, H., Auber, R.E. and Herman, W.H., (1998). Global burden of diabetes, 1995–2025: prevalence, numerical estimates, and projections. Diabetes Care. 21 (9), 1414–31.

Klein, S., Sheard, N.F, Pi-Sunyer, X, Daly, A., Wylie-Rosett, J., Kulkarni, K. and Clark N.G.. (2004). Weight management through lifestyle modification for the prevention and management of type 2 diabetes: rationale and strategies. A statement of the American Diabetes Association, the North American Association for the Study of Obesity, and the American Society for Clinical Nutrition. *The American Journal of clinical nutrition*. 80 (1), p257–263.

Kozłowska, L., Rydzewski, A., Fiderkiewicz, B., Wasińska-Krawczyk, A., Grzechnik, A. and Rosołowska-Huszcz D.. (2010). Adiponectin, Resistin and Leptin Response to Dietary Intervention in Diabetic Nephropathy. Journal of Renal Nutrition. 10 (1)

Life Clinic International. (2010). Advances in Diabetes. Available: http://www.lifeclinic.com/focus/diabetes/advances.asp Top. Last accessed 15 June 2010.

Liu, R., Bal, H.S., Desta, T., Behl, Y. and Graves, D.T.. (2006). Tumor Necrosis Factor-Mediates Diabetes-Enhanced Apoptosis of Matrix-Producing Cells and Impairs Diabetic Healing. *American Journal of Pathology.* 168 (1), p757–764.

Lund, S.S., Tarnow, L., Frandsen, M., Nielsen, B.B., Hansen, B.V., Pedersen, O., Parving, H., and Vaag, A.A.. (2009). Combining insulin with metformin or an insulin secretagogue in non-obese patients with type 2 diabetes:12 month, randomised, double blind trial.. *British Medical Journal.* 339 (b4324), p1–11.

Nauck, A.M., Berria, R., Ratner, R.E., Boldrin, M., Kapitza, C., and Balena, R. (2009). Treatment With the Human Once-Weekly Glucagon-Like Peptide-1 Analog Taspoglutide in Combination With Metformin Improves Glycemic Control and Lowers Body Weight in Patients With Type 2 Diabetes Inadequately Controlled With Metformin Alone. *Journal of Diabetes Care.* 32 (7), p1237–1243.

Orozco, L.J., Buchleitner, A.M., Gimenez-Perez, G., Roqué i Figuls, M., Richter, B. and Mauricio, D.. (2008). Exercise or exercise and diet for preventing type 2 diabetes. The Cochrane library. 1 (3), p1–82.

Reasner, C.A.. (1999). Promising new approaches.Diabetes, *Obesity and Metabolism.* 14 (1), p41–48.

Rosenstock, J., Sugimoto, D., Stewart, A.J., Soltes-RAK, E., Strange, P., and Dailey, G. (2006). Triple Therapy in Type 2 Diabetes Insulin glargine or rosiglitazone added to combination therapy of sulfonylurea plus metformin in insulin-naïve patients. *Journal of Diabetes Care.* 29 (3), 2006.

Scheen, A.J., Finer, N., Hollander, P., Jensen, M.D., and Van Gaal, L.F.. (2006). Efficacy and tolerability of rimonabant in overweight or obese patients with type 2 diabetes: a randomised controlled study.. *The Lancet.* 368 (9548), p1660–1672.

Shulman, G.I., and Lowell, B.B.. (2010). Mitochondrial Dysfunction and Type 2 Diabetes. *Journal of science.* 307 (3), p384–387.

Stenlof, K., Rossner, S., Vercruysse, F., Kumar, A., Fitchet, M., and Sjostrom, L.. (2007). Topiramate in the treatment of obese subjects with drug-naive type 2 diabetes.. *Diabetes, Obesity and Metabolism.* 9 (2), p360–368.

Steyn, N.P., Mann, J., and Bennett, P.H.. (2004). Diet, Nutrition and the Prevention of Type 2 Diabetes.. Public Health Nutrition. 7 (1A), p147–165.

Thomas, D., Elliott, E.J. and Naughton, G.A.. (2009). Exercise for type 2 diabetes mellitus (Review). The Cochrane Library. 1 (1), p1–53.

Tzoulaki, I., Molokhia, M., Curcin, V., Little, M.P., Millett, C.J., Ng, A., Hughes, R.I., Khunti, K., Wilkins, M.R., Majeed, A., and Elliott, P.. (2009). Risk of cardiovascular disease and all cause mortality among patients with type 2 diabetes prescribed oral antidiabetes drugs: retrospective cohort study using UK general practice research database.. British Medical Journal. 339 (b4731), p1–9.

Weisberg, S.P., McCann, D., Desai, M., Rosenbaum, M., Leibel, R.L., and Ferrante, A.W.. (2003). Obesity is associated with macrophage accumulation in adipose tissue. The Journal for Clinical Investigation. 112 (12), p1796–1808

Wild, S., Roglic, G., Green, A., Sicree, R., and King, H.. (2004). Global Prevalence of Diabetes. Estimates for the year 2000 and projections for 2030.. Diabetes Care. 27 (5), p1047–1053.

Williamson, D.A., Rejeski, J., Lang, W., Van Dorsten, B., Fabricatore, A.N. and Toledo, K.. (2009). Impact of a Weight Management Program on Health-Related Quality of Liffe in Overweight Adults with Type 2 Diabetes. Archinternmed. 169 (2), p163–171.

Wulffele, M.G., Kooy, A., Lehert P., Betts, D., Ogterop, J.C., Van der Burg, B.B., Donker, A.J.M., and Stehouwer, C.D.A. (2002). Combination of Insulin and Metformin in the Treatment of Type 2 Diabetes. Diabetes Care. 25 (12), p2133–2140.

2

THE EXPERIENCE BREATHLESSNESS IN ADULTS 'ASTHMA PATIENTS'

Johnson Mbabazi and Mohammed Sattar

ABSTRACT

This research helps add knowledge on breathlessness in adults diagnosed with 'asthma thus 'asthma patients'. Many elderly patients across the world experience shortness of breathe also known as dyspnoea. This book aims at answering the what, why, how questions following patient experience and how respiratory clinical team manage the condition. It also helps explain and shows the similarities and differences between actual patient experiences with that of the literature. This research will also respiratory clinicians understand what patient experience with chronic asthma. It also helps patients understand interventions needed in management the condition. It is evident that breathlessness is a major challenge to asthma patients. Breathing exercises minimise Shortness of Breath and care in elderly is mainly palliative and supervision. Medical interventions include; nebulisers, nebusal and oxygen. Posture (Sitting up right) supports elderly breathing without causing much stress. Physical interventions including; breathing exercises may complement medical treatment are so helpful to reduce breathing discomfort. Lastly, adjusting patient activities to his abilities like washing, dressing, walking helps promote their autonomy and their personal development in the activities of daily living.

AIMS AND OBJECTIVES

- Asthma and its relation to breathlessness
- Causes of breathlessness in an asthma patient
- Patient experience
- Patient experiences verses literature
- Patient management by clinical practitioners (respiratory team)
- Interventions by clinical practitioners (respiratory team)
- Conclusion
- References

THREE MAIN SECTIONS

1. Patient experience
   - What, why, how

2. Patient vs literature
   - What, why, how
3. Patient compared with patients
   - What, why how

INTRODUCTION OF ASTHMA AS A CONDITION

- Asthma is a chronic inflammatory lung disease that narrows the airways
- Mainly characterised by breathlessness

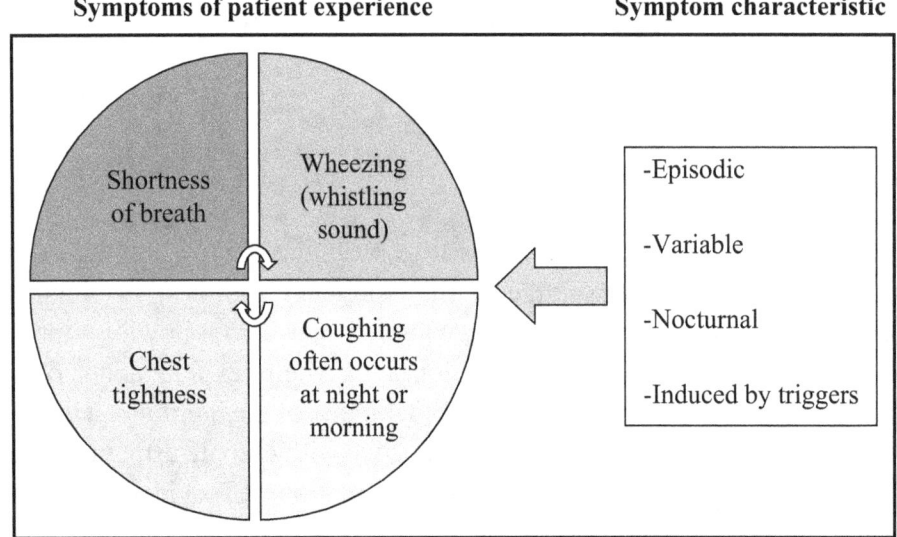

COMMON TRIGGERS OF ASTHMA

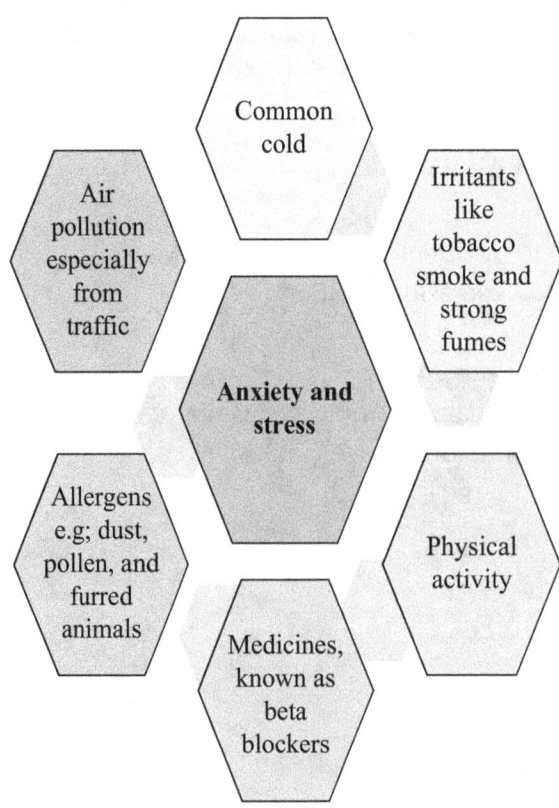

SHORTNESS OF BREATH

- Shortness of breath is defined as a "subjective experience of breathing discomfort." Along with cough, wheeze, and chest tightness, it is a typical symptom of asthma.
- In asthma, shortness of breath is usually caused by the narrowing of the airways. The airways become narrow for one or both reasons:
  - The muscles that surround the airways tighten up ("bronchospasm").
  - Inflammation makes the airways swell and fill with mucus.
- The medical term for shortness of breath is dyspnoea. People describe it as air hunger, fast breathing, running out of air, or not being able to breathe fast or deep enough. Similar to thirst, hunger, or pain, it is nearly impossible to ignore. Because it is a subjective symptom, you can feel and describe it, but a health care provider cannot observe or measure it.
- Some breathlessness is normal, such as after hard exercising or when you have a stuffy nose. However, it is a problem when it is greater than expected for a given level of physical effort.
- If shortness of breath continues for more than a month, it is considered chronic. Shortness of breath also can come on suddenly. Breathlessness is a symptom of many different conditions, so your medical history and a physical examination will provide important clues to the cause. For about two-thirds of patients, the signs and symptoms are enough to make an accurate diagnosis. Occasionally, additional tests may be needed.

WHAT OTHER CONDITIONS CAN CAUSE SHORTNESS OF BREATH?

- In adults, asthma, congestive heart failure, heart attack, chronic obstructive pulmonary disease, scarring of the lung tissue, and anxiety cause 85% of shortness of breath cases. More than one-third of people have two or more causes of breathlessness. The occurrence of breathlessness is highest in people who are 55 to 69 years old.

EXAMPLES OF QUESTIONS TO ASK WITH SHORTNESS OF BREATH

- When did you first feel short of breath?
- How long has it been going on?
- How would you describe it?
- How severe is the feeling of breathlessness?
- Is it more difficult to get air in or out?
- Do you feel this way all the time, or does it come and go?
- What other symptoms have you noticed?
- Breathlessness that comes and goes is a sign of asthma. Shortness of breath caused by allergies or other common asthma triggers is another sign of asthma. Finally, breathlessness with wheezing indicates asthma.
- If the history and physical exam suggest that you have asthma, your provider may asked you to do spirometry. Spirometry is an important lung function test to evaluate how much and how quickly you can exhale air. The test is usually done before and after taking a medication that opens the airways ("bronchodilator"). Asthma is likely if medications are able to open the airways.

HOW IS ASTHMA-RELATED SHORTNESS OF BREATH TREATED?

- If shortness of breath is due to intermittent asthma, your provider may prescribe a rescue inhaler for use as needed. Asthma is considered intermittent if symptoms occur less than three days per week, do not limit activities, and rarely wake you up at night.
- If shortness of breath and other symptoms occur more frequently, your provider may recommend starting long-term treatment for asthma. Initial treatment of persistent asthma usually involves inhaled corticosteroids and avoiding asthma triggers.
- For some people asthma, breathlessness and being out of shape become a vicious cycle. Exercise is a common trigger for asthma symptoms. These symptoms can be uncomfortable, which discourages people from exercising. Unfortunately, getting out of shape makes you feel even more short of breath when you are active. Your provider can work with you to find the right combination of medications that allows you to be active. Your provider or respiratory therapist can work with you to make an exercise plan.

CASE STUDY

Patient history

- 85 year old male with multiple conditions
- Such as Heart failure, acute kidney injury & asthma
- Patient's asthma was diagnosed as late onset
- Anxiety and stress in chewing food and swallowing dysfunction

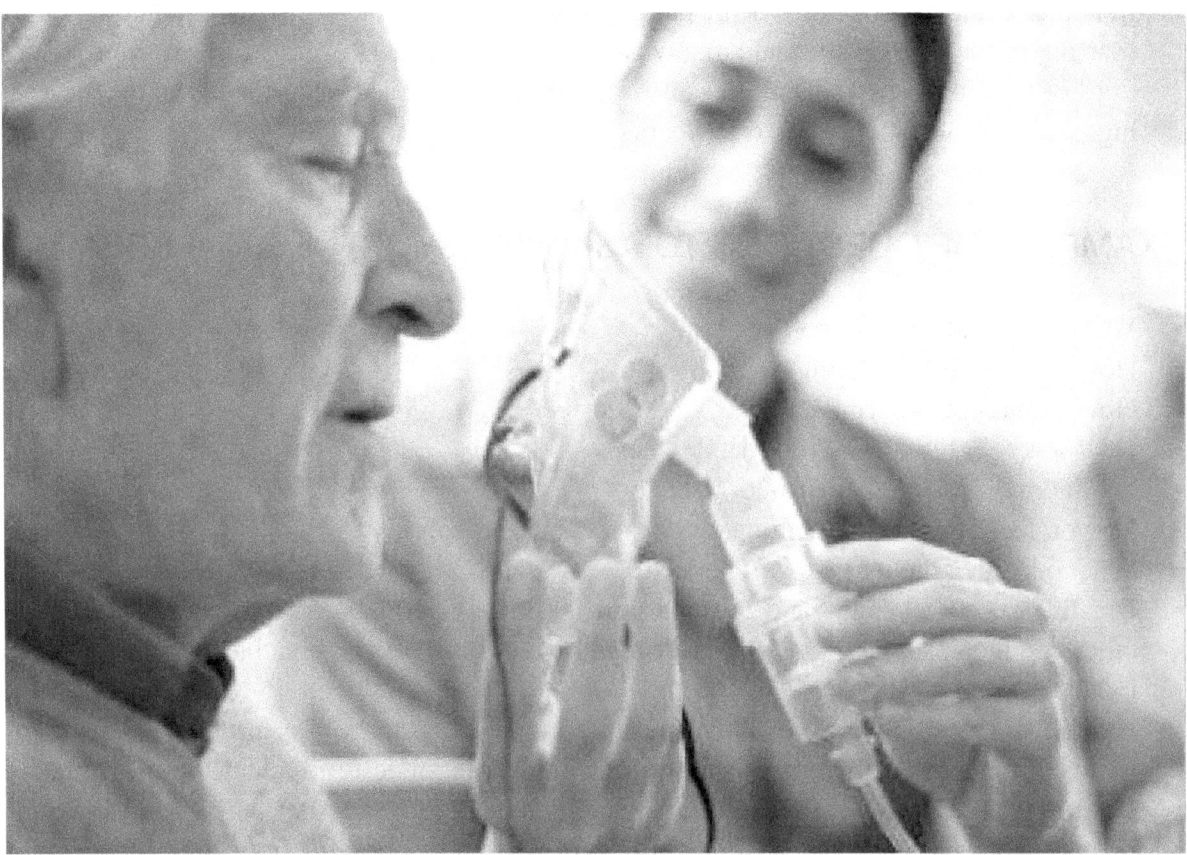

Google image, 2018

PATIENT EXPERIENCE

- Breathlessness in speech and mobility
- Patient stopped playing cricket and badminton due to asthma
- Patient sleeps well during day but runs out of breath during night
- Patient worried about too much care from relatives
- Worried of the amount of medication the patient takes

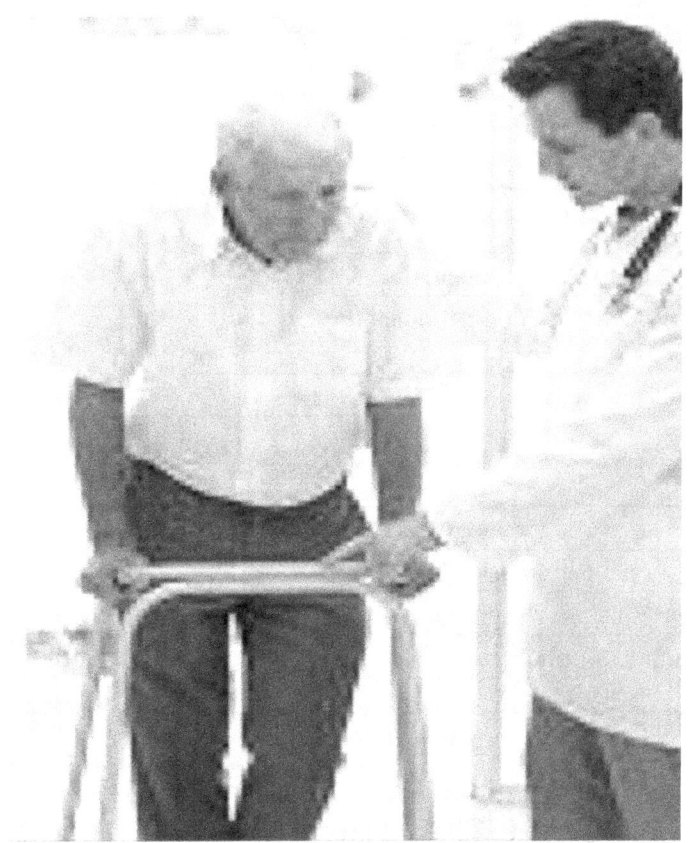

Google image, 2017

KEY CHALLENGES TO THE PATIENT

Breathing	Shortness of breath (SoB) during night
Loss of breath under stress	Speaking
Eating, drinking and swallowing blocks airway	Mobility: Uses Zimmer frame & walks few steps feels breathless

SEARCH STRATEGY

CINAHL

Search term	Number of hits
1) patient* experience* or patient* satisfaction	50
2) AND Breathless* or dyspnea or dyspnoea	
3) AND Asthma* or chronic obstruction pulmonary diseases or COPD	
1, 2, 3 add subject age 80 and over	18

MEDLINE

Search term	Number of hits
1) patient* experience* or patient* satisfaction	96
2) AND Breathless* or dyspnea or dyspnoea	
3) AND Asthma* or chronic obstruction pulmonary diseases or COPD	
1, 2, 3 add subject age 80 and over	14

BRITISH NURSING INDEX

Search term	Number of hits
1) patient* experience* or patient* satisfaction	28
2) AND Breathless* or dyspnea or dyspnoea	
3) AND Asthma* or chronic obstruction pulmonary diseases or COPD	
1, 2, 3 add subject age 80 and over	7

PATIENT EXPERIENCE VS LITERATURE

	Breathlessness among the elderly						
Study	Participants Gender and age	Summary characteristics of participants	Research design	Research method	Intervention Physical, Medical & psychological	Main findings	Similarities/ differences literature with patient experience
Dirks et al, 2007 Dyspnoea in Asthmatics: Qualitative Descriptors vs Quantitative Perception	587 asthmatics (f = 396, m = 191, 65–84 yrs)	-Partial breathlessness -Strenuous breathing -No deep breaths -Tight chest	Prospective observational study	Qualitative research studies -Dyspnoea questionnaire	Breathlessness; -At rest -Paced walking -Climbing stairs	Breathlessness with; -Walking fast -dressing -And/or undressing	The findings are; -comparable to presented case -Patient challenges common to others

(*Continued*)

| Leupoldt and Dahme, 2007 Review Dyspnoea in COPD: Psychological aspects | 42 asthmatics (f=8, m=14 μ=86 yrs) | patients with COPD took part in the program that offered several modules of patient education, self-monitoring, training instructions and patient encouragement via the Internet | Prospective observational study | Different methods Questionnarie, observational study -Patient education methods, focusing on behavioural changes. | -↓ dyspnoea > 3 months. Educational breathing techniques; -Abdominal -pursed lip -nasal breathing | 3-month patients ↓dyspnoea during activities of daily life and increased self-efficacy in managing their symptoms. | -Different psychological and behavioural interventions reduce comorbid psychological disorders hence improve the perception of SoB. -Future studies are needed to show these findings & to provide more detailed insights into the psychological aspects on perception of SoB in COPD. Agrees with my findings (Behaviour cognitive therapy). |

ROPER LOGAN AND TIERNEY'S MODEL

Patient main issues

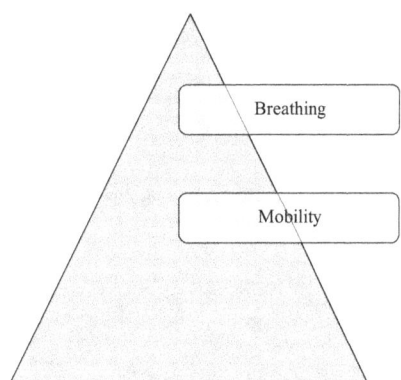

Holistic model

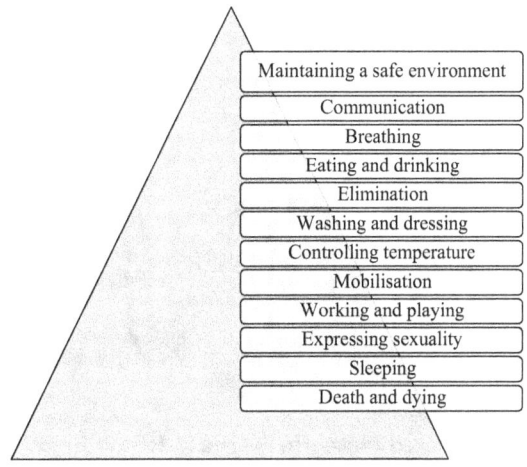

Roper, Logan, and Tierney 2018

Roper, Logan, and Tierney 2018 model

- Assess the patient's relative independence in performing activities
- Nurse in formulating individualised care plans aimed at increasing independence

INTERVENTION BY CLINICAL RESPIRATORY TEAM

Physical

Pulmonary rehabilitation

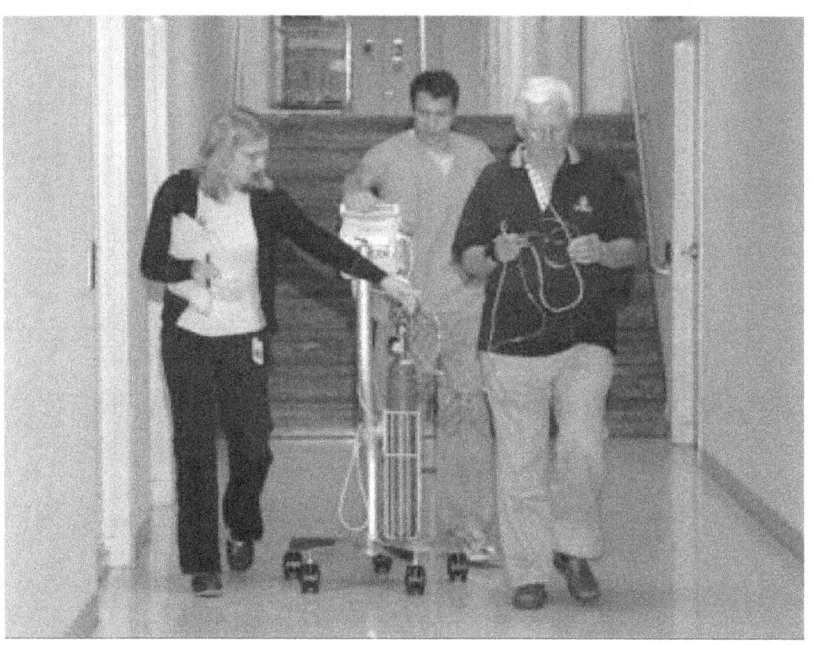

Breathless exercises

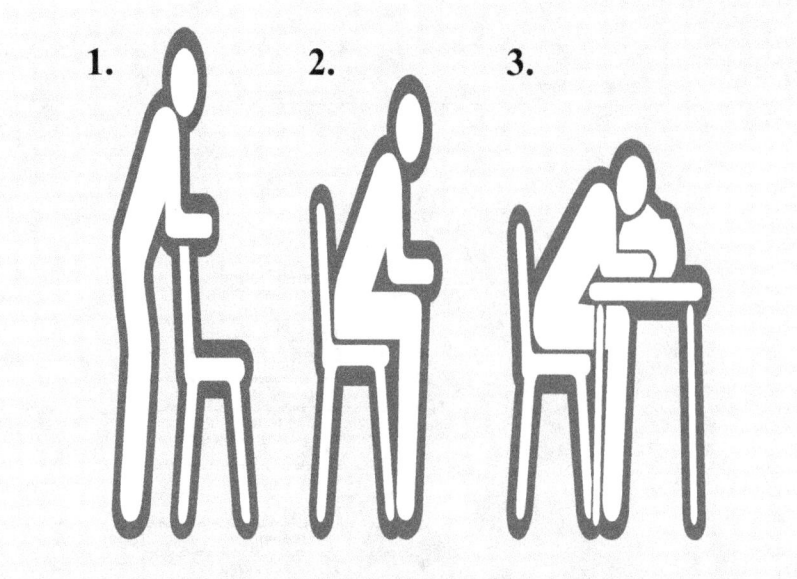

Association for Chartered Physiotherapists in Respiratory Care (ACPRC), 2015

Medical

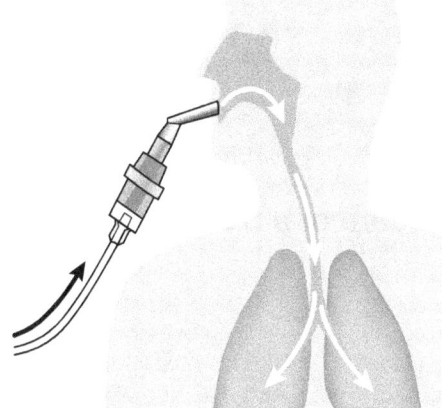

Nebulisers open up airways (Salbutamol)

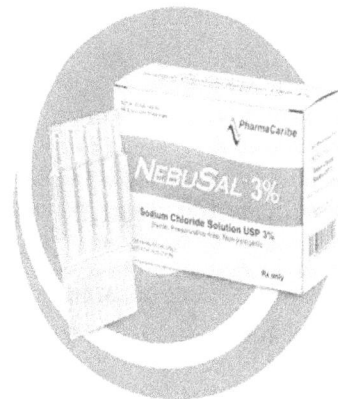

Help with sputum (nebusal)

Oxygen for home

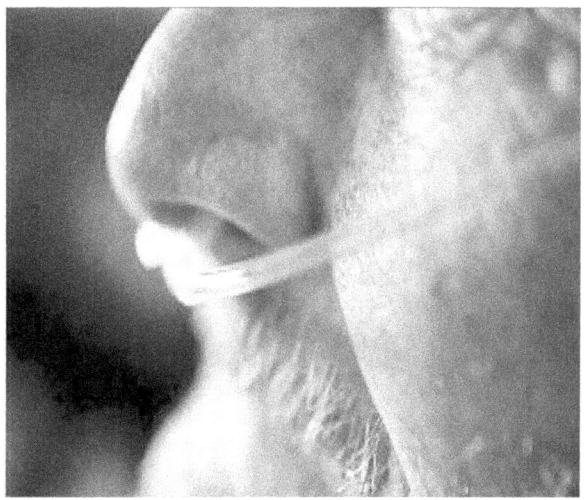

CONCEPTUAL MODEL

A composition of concepts which is used to help a breathless patient experience and understand the role of a respiratory team.

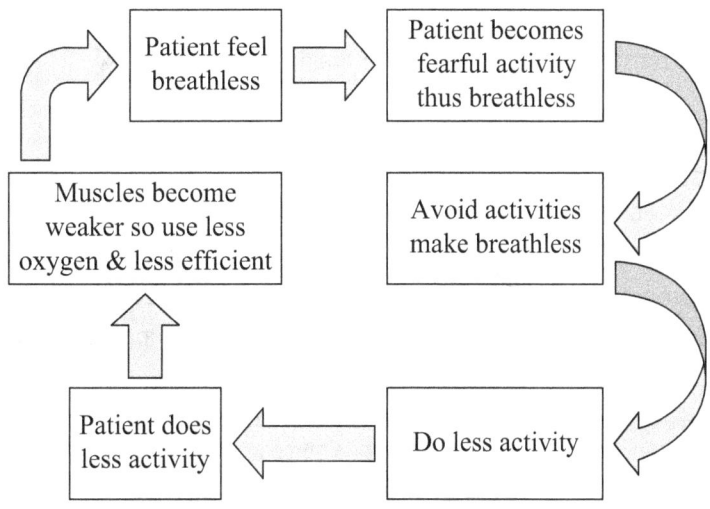

AVAILABLE PATIENT SUPPORT

- Government funding (NHS 2015)
- Social workers
- Domestic carers
- Community nurses

Challenges a respiratory team may face in care of a patient

- Managing emotion aspect of anxiety
- Unpredictable asthma attacks
- Medications
- Infections
- Morbidity & Cognition Behaviour Therapy

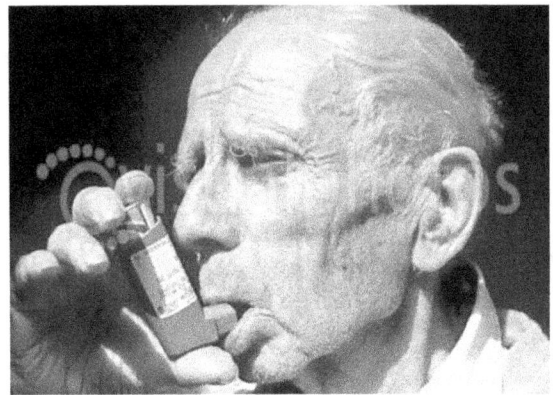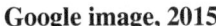
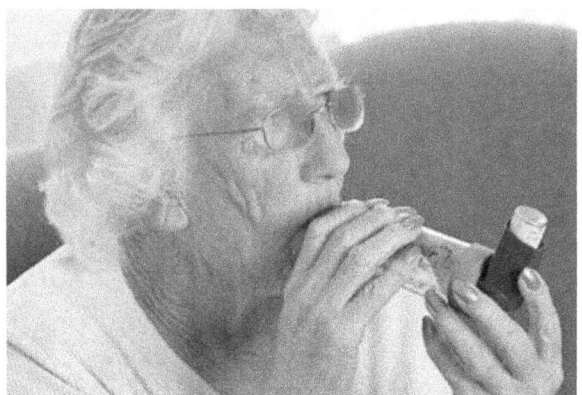

Google image, 2015   **Google image, 2016**

CONCLUSION AND RECOMMENDATIONS

- Breathlessness is a major challenge to asthma patients
- Breathing exercises minimise Shortness of Breath
- Care is mainly palliative and supervision
- Medical interventions include; nebulisers, nebusal and oxygen
- Posture (Sitting up right)
- Physical interventions including; breathing exercises may complement medical treatment
- Adjusting patient activities to his abilities like washing, dressing, walking

ACKNOWLEDGEMENT AND DEDICATION

I (Mr. Johnson Mbabazi FRSPH) would like to acknowledge all the respiratory team I worked with on Granby ward in Harrogate Hospital that helped me carryout this research. In addition thank the asthmatic elderly patients that let me understand their asthma experience. I would like above all thank particularly Stewart Pearson ward manager would gave me consent carryout this research. Dr. Mohammad would like to dedicate this palliative clinical research to all asthmatic patients suffering breathlessness in his surgery and globally. This research is dedicated to all those suffering asthma globally and I know this research will help anyone manage his or her symptoms.

REFERENCES

Association for Chartered Physiotherapists in Respiratory. (2015). The Association of Physiotherapy in Respiratory Care. The ACPRC publish a Journal annually, a monthly E- Newsletter, and an Electronic biannual Respiratory Review. 12 (1), 1–15.

Dirks J.F, Schraa J.C, and Robinson, S.K. (2007). Patient mislabelling of symptoms: implications for patient-physician communication and medical outcome. International Journal Psychiatry Medicine. 27 (7), p15–27.

Googleimage. (2016). Daily Wellness; Wordpress. Available: http://www.dailywellness.net/category/asthma/. Last accessed Accessed 14 July 2016.

Googleimage. (2018). PharmaCaribe. Available: http://pharmacaribe.com/ourproducts/nebusal-3/. Last accessed 14th July 2018.

Googleimage. (2016). Elderly man using an aerosol inhaler for asthma. Available: https://www.google.co.uk/search?q=breathlessness+asthma+elderly&biw=1280&bih=907&source=lnms&tbm=isch&sa=X&ved=0CAYQ_AUoAWoVChMItOePlabaxgIVSdcUCh1xbAiX&dpr=1#tbm=isch&q=+asthma+elderly&imgrc=h0Y64V17. Last accessed 14th July 2016

Leupoldt and Dahme. (2007). Psychological aspects in the perception of dyspnea in obstructive pulmonary diseases. Review journal of respiratory medicine. 12 (2), p418–425.

Pechmann, C. (2015). Development of a Twitter-Based Intervention for Smoking Cessation that Encourages High-Quality Social Media Interactions via Auto messages. Journal of Medical Internet Research. 17 (2), p1–6.

Roper N., Logan, W and Tierney, A.J. (2018). The Roper-Logan-Tierney Model of Nursing: Based on Activities of Living. Journal of Advanced Nursing. 69 (1), p21–35.

3

EPIDEMIOLOGICAL REFERENCE BOOK OF CERVICAL CANCER

Johnson Mbabazi

ABSTRACT

This reference book explains that cervical screening checks the health of your cervix. It's not a test for cancer, it's a test to help prevent cancer. It additionally, helps clinicians, public health specialist, health promotional specialists and individuals develop epidemiological understanding of cervical cancer. More importantly, develop an understanding and awareness on the importance of early cervical cancer screening on current approaches, policies and campaigns in relation to new cervical cancer campaigns. Lastly, cervical cancer screen will help detect abnormal cell changes in a woman's cervix but if left untreated, this could turn into cancer. This is because some types of Human papillomavirus (HPV) can lead to cell changes in your cervix and cancer.

AIMS AND OBJECTIVES

- To develop epidemiological understanding of cervical cancer screening
- To develop an understanding and awareness on the importance of early cervical cancer screening
- Current approaches, policies and campaigns in relation to new cervical cancer campaigns

INTRODUCTION

"Epidemiology is the study of the distribution and determinants of disease in human populations" (Barker and Rose, 1984 p 5).

This report examines the epidemiology of cervical cancer in the UK. It does so by critically analysing and evaluating current literature (journals and newspaper articles) on cervical cancer and examines the prevalence, incidence, causal relations, risk factors and determinants with evidence of the threat to health.

In addition, the report includes a discussion of the implications of the lay epidemiology and media representations of the cervical cancer risk.

A critique of current solutions to the cervical cancer problem and possible evidence-based changes to the current strategy is then made.

Facts of cervical cancer

1. Worldwide, cervical cancer is the third most common cancer among women
2. Worldwide, every two minutes a woman dies from cervical cancer
3. 86% of cervical cancer cases and 88% of deaths occur in developing regions
4. In India, cervical cancer is the single most common cancer
5. For every 35 women in India, one will be diagnosed with cervical cancer
6. In the United States, one in every 192 women will develop cervical cancer
7. Sexually transmitted HPV is a necessary factor in cervical cancer
8. Worldwide, 70% of cervical cancer is caused by HPV types 16 and 18
9. More than 80% of women will be infected with HPV at some time
10. Cervical cancer is one of three cancers effectively prevented with screening

Symptoms of cervical cancer

Common symptoms of cervical cancer can include:

- Heavier periods than you normally have
- Vaginal bleeding between periods
- Vaginal bleeding after sex
- Vaginal bleeding after the menopause (after you have stopped having periods)

Other symptoms include:

- A smelly vaginal discharge
- urine infections that keep coming back
- Pain in the lower tummy or back
- Very early-stage cervical cancer may not cause any symptoms. It is usually found and treated because of cervical screening tests

New Cervical campaign /main purpose

- A new drive to ensure General Practitioners spot cervical cancer symptoms earlier in young women and refer patients correctly.
- The Campaign was with independent Advisory Committee on Cervical Screening (ACCS). An awareness campaign for General Practioners, Health promotional specialist and practice nurses.
- An audit of all young women diagnosed with cervical cancer looking at their symptoms before diagnosis.
- An expansion of work to increase screening uptake in women aged 25 to 34 ensure early detection.

NATURE OF CERVICAL CANCER

"Cervical cancer is a malignant neoplasm arising from the uterine cervix"
(Martin-Hirsch, 2011).

It is a malignant growth of either the glandular cells or the squamous cells which make up the cervix caused mainly by Human papillomavirus (HPV). HPV has been identified as the main cause of Intensive Cervical Cancer (ICC) with at least 13 different strains related to ICC (Cogliano et al, 2005). These 13 are only a subset of over 100 known HPV strains which 80% of women contract at some point in their lives (Ault, 2007). Consequently, cervical cancer is quite difficult to prevent and control.

When it affects the squamous cells, cervical cancer is known as squamous cell cancer (SCC) which accounts for about 90% of all ICC cases. The other 10% of ICC cases are adenocarcinomas and occur in cervical glandular cells. This difference in frequency occurs because the flat thin squamous cells, being surface cells (Ectocervix and close to the vagina), are the primary site for HPV virus infection and are more susceptible compared to the cells that make up the glands.

Incidence, mortality, and aetiology of cervical cancer

Global Trends Despite the availability of effective methods for prevention, cervical cancer is the third most common cancer among women worldwide and the seventh most common cancer overall. In many economically developing regions of the world, including Africa, Asia, South and Central America, and parts of the Pacific region, cervical cancer is the single most common cancer among women with an age standardised rate (ASR) ranging from 30 per 100,000 women in parts of Eastern and Western Africa to 24.6 per 100,000 women in South-Central Asia. In 2008 there were an estimated 530,000 incident cases and 275,000 associated mortalities.

Current data suggest that of the total global burden, 86 percent of all cervical cancer diagnoses and 88 percent of associated mortalities occur among women living in economically developing regions of the world. In addition to significant disparities in the actual incidence of cervical cancer between countries, substantial differences in the overall contribution of cervical cancer to total cancer burden also exist.

In many economically developing countries, cervical cancer represents 13 percent of all females cancers compared to less than six percent in other regions of the world.14

Observed disparities in cervical cancer incidence and mortality are largely accounted for by inequities in cervical cancer screening. In countries with well-organised screening programs, rates of cervical cancer morbidity and mortality have declined significantly over the past several decades.

However, in many economically 18 developing countries where cervical cancer is not recognized as a public health priority and screening programs are mostly opportunistic, the incidence of cervical cancer remains unchanged, and in several cases continues to increase.

Prevalence of Cervical Cancer

"Prevalence of a disease is defined as the number of affected persons present in the population at a specific time divided by the number of persons in the population at that time" (Gordis, 1996, p. 32).

Table 1 shows the one, five and ten year prevalence for cervical cancer in the UK at the end of 2006. This figure is from the Office of National Statistics (ONS), which is the UK statistics authority, capturing primary data through multiple reliable sources across all the four countries in the UK. It

Table 1. Cervical cancer prevalence in the UK, at 31st December 2006

	1 year prevalence	5 year prevalence	10 year prevalence
Females	2,517	10,125	19,046

Office of National Statistics, 2011.

can be seen that in December 2006, over 19,000 women in the UK had survived cervical cancer for over 10 years post-diagnosis.

It is argued that early detection, more extensive screening, better awareness, vaccination and otherwise improving public health interventions means more people are living longer post-diagnosis and that this will be reflected in the 15 year prevalence for December 2011.

Incidence of Cervical Cancer

"Incidence of a disease is defined as the number of new cases of the disease that occur during a specified period of time in a population at risk for developing the disease" (Gordis, 1996, p. 31).

In 2007, there were over 2830 new cases of cervical cancer diagnosed in the UK (National Cancer Intelligence Network (NCIN), 2008).

How these were age-related can be seen in Figure 1 below. This information was collated by the NCIN which is the main UK initiative embedded directly within the NHS that collects complete first hand data on all cancer cases and acts as the main NHS-wide repository for all cancer statistics and research, including cervical cancer. It operates a database and web-reporting tool called the UK Cancer Information Service (UKCIS) which provides secure, timely and reliable primary data on all aspects of cancer across the UK.

Cervical cancer is more common in younger women, with half of the cases occurring in women under 50, and it is the most prevalent cancer in women under 35. This is mainly linked to sexual activity and HPV transmission.

The Incidence rate is maximum for women between 30 and 39, after which it falls steadily to peak again in women over 70. The high incidence in women over 70 can be explained by a cohort effect relating to those born before cervical screening got rolled out by the NHS.

The cervical screening programme which began in 1989 and which has now achieved a high penetration in the UK, has helped reduce the incidence of cervical cancer as seen in Figure 2 below. In the last ten years, the incidence of ICC has fallen by 10%.

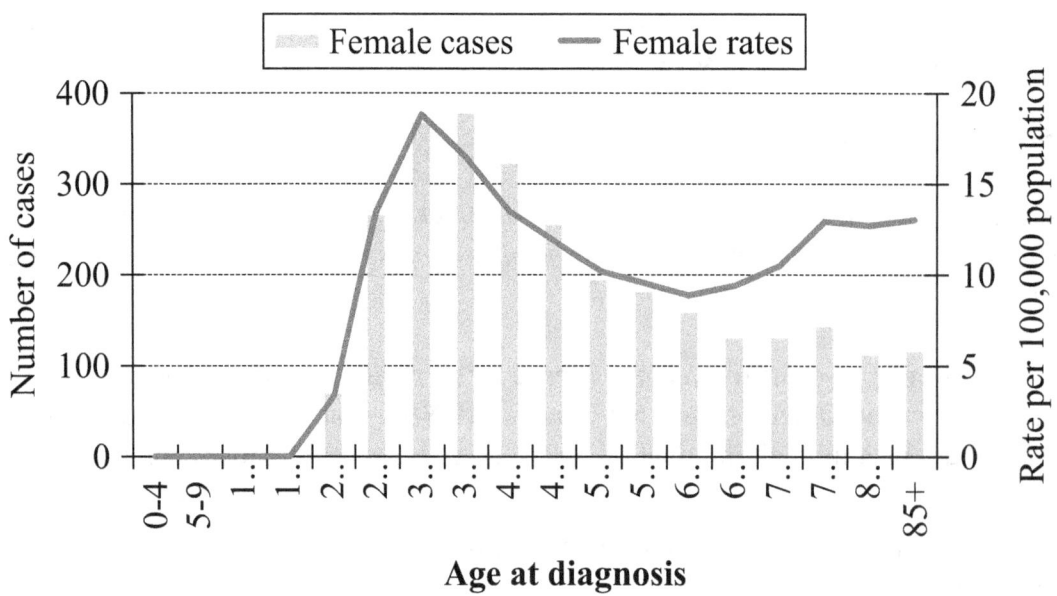

(National Cancer Intelligence Network, 2011).

Figure 1. Numbers of new cases and age specific incidence rates, by sex, cervical cancer, UK 2007.

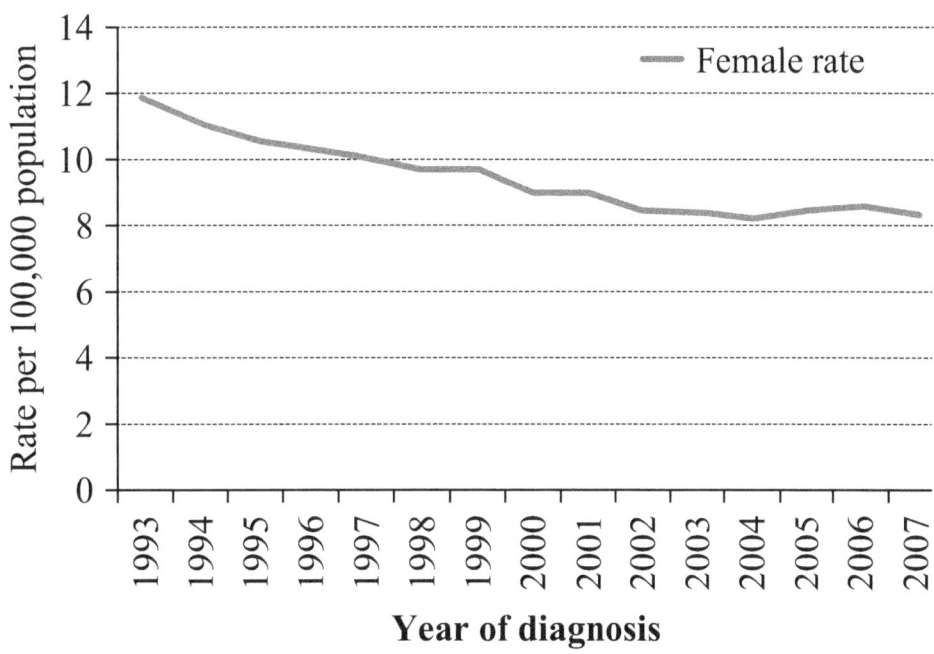

(National Cancer Intelligence Network, 2011)

Figure 2. Age standardised incidence rates, cervical cancer, UK, 1993–2007.

Regular screening means early detection and when cervical cancer is detected in the early stages, the chances of a full recovery are higher.

Causal relationships, risk factors and determinants

Cervical cancer is mainly caused by HPV, although several other factors are known to increase the likelihood of ICC. These include smoking, family history and infection with other sexually transmitted diseases (STDs) like herpes or Chlamydia. Human Immunodeficiency Virus (HIV) sufferers and women on contraceptive pills long term also face an increased risk.

It is, however, still unclear why HPV infection leads to ICC in some cases and not in others. This is of critical interest to researchers, as being able to narrow down which cases will develop to ICC will greatly reduce treatment costs for the NHS. Currently, all infected women showing CIN-3 or severe abnormalities in cervical cells are treated, even though not all would progress into ICC.

The interplay of host, agent and environment makes it appropriate to use Mausner and Bahns triangle of causations model from all existing models to summarise the causal relationships for cervical cancer as shown in Figure 3 below.

Cervical cancer is a transmissible infectious disease resulting from the interaction of a host (women), a disease causing agent (13 known strains of HPV) and the environment (social and physical which promotes exposure and susceptibility) which can best be examined using the components of this epidemiological triangle (Gordis, 1996).

This means that the disease can be prevented as well as cured. The former, by procedures and behaviours that prevent exposure and reduce susceptibility, and the latter by those that attack the agent.

Socio-economic status has been linked to an increased cervical cancer risk. Analysed to Carstairs deprivation scores (A scale of material deprivation designed using four census variables – lack of car ownership, household overcrowding, low social class and male unemployment.), cervical cancer incidence and mortality can be shown to increase with increasing deprivation as seen in Figure 4 below.

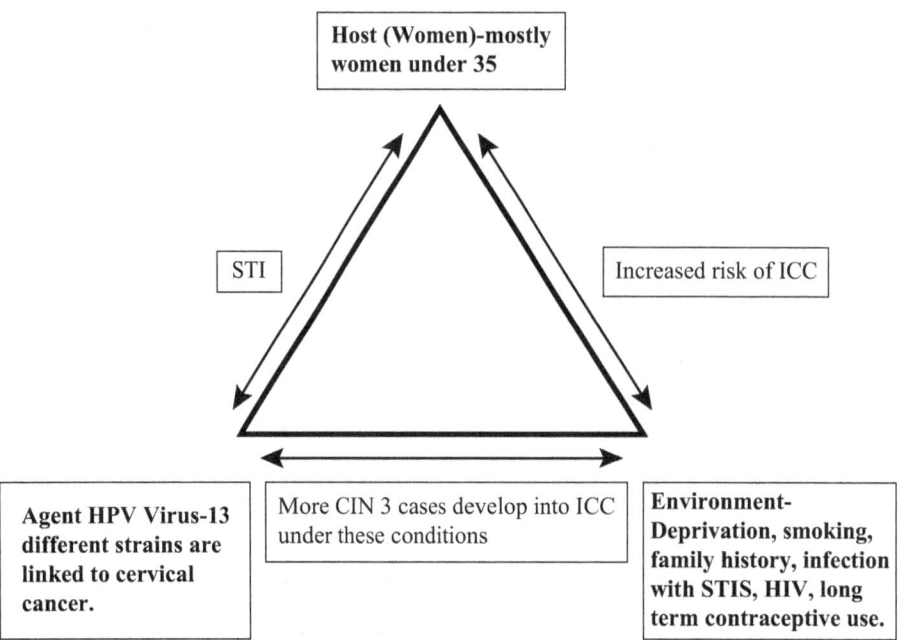

Triangle of causation (adapted from Mausner and Bahn, 1985).

Figure 3. Epidemiological Triangle of causations for cervical cancer adopted from Mausner and Bahn, 1985.

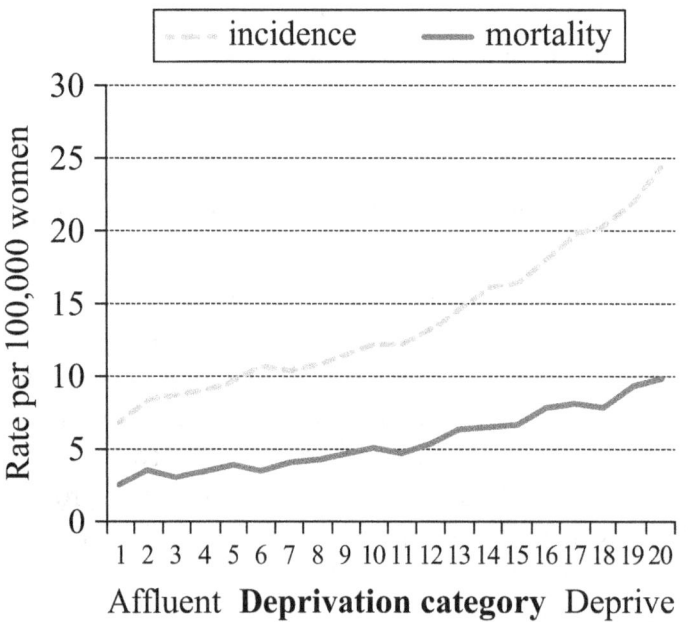

(National Cancer Intelligence Network, 2011).

Figure 4. Age-standardised incidence of and mortality due to cervical cancer by deprivation category, England and Wales, 1990–93.

The most deprived women are several times more likely to develop cervical cancer.

Determinants of health are any of five main factors that contribute to a person's health. These include genes and biology, health behaviours, social environment, physical environment and access to medical care. For cervical cancer specifically, these can be developed to include: age, sex, fitness, socio-economic status, medical history (HIV, STDs and family history) and behaviours such as smoking, unprotected sexual activity and an extended use of contraceptive pills amongst others.

Examining the determinants of cervical cancer in this way highlights the importance of social, economic and behavioural contributions to cervical cancer. This means that by impacting these positively through public health interventions, cervical cancer can be prevented. On the other hand, it can also be argued that the causes of cervical cancer are portrayed in such a way that the impact of individual choice appears limited.

Evidence of the threat to health

The foregoing prevalence, incidence and causal relationships give perspective to the cervical cancer problem and inform on the relevance of its threat to health.

Roughly 2,700 women are diagnosed yearly with cervical cancer, accounting for about 2% of cancers in women. However, it is very common in women under 35, second only to lung cancer in this age bracket (ONS, 2010).

Unfortunately, the last six years have seen government agencies and policy informers, pressured by pharmaceutical companies into alarming the UK government with health scare tactics, in a bid to sell their patented drugs and vaccines.

Both the bird and swine flu campaigns of 2006 and 2009 respectively are examples of such alarms. The outbreak of swine flu in particular was portrayed as a pandemic which could wipe out millions and resulted in the large scale procurement and stocking of Tamiflu, which in retrospect was an overkill as infections in the UK ranged in the hundreds (WHO, 2009).

It is therefore, highly important to weigh the evidence of the threat to public health in a balanced and unbiased way. This can be done by investigating mortality and survival rates and both direct and indirect (infertility for example) costs of cervical cancer.

Research into prevention of cervical cancer

HPV vaccines

Vaccines, such as Cervarix and Gardasil, have been developed to prevent HPV infection. There are many different HPV strains. HPV types 16 and 18 are known to increase the risk of cervical cancer.

Several research trials have tested vaccines as a way of preventing infection with HPV. The trials have shown that the vaccines help to prevent abnormal changes in the cervix that may develop into cancer. In the UK, HPV vaccination is offered in school to all girls aged 12 to 13.

Research suggests that this vaccination programme will greatly lower the number of cases of cervical cancer. It will also reduce the need for colposcopy.

Researchers are looking at a type of magnetic resonance imaging (MRI) scan called diffusion weighted MRI for cervical cancer. The aim of this study is to find out if the diffusion weighted MRI can show whether cervical cancer is likely to have a good or a bad outcome.

Surgery

Surgery is the usual treatment for early stage cervical cancer.

- Surgery for early cervical cancer

Researchers are looking at different ways of doing surgery for early cervical cancer. They are comparing removal of the womb and cervix (a simple hysterectomy) with the usual treatment (a radical hysterectomy).

A radical hysterectomy involves removing:

- the womb (including the cervix)
- all the tissues holding the womb in place
- the top of the vagina
- all the lymph nodes around the womb

The trial wants to find out if a simple hysterectomy is as good as a radical hysterectomy in treating cervical cancer. It also wants to check if the simple hysterectomy gives fewer side effects and a better quality of life after the surgery.

Chemotherapy

Researchers are:

Comparing chemotherapy before surgery with chemotherapy and radiotherapy (chemo radiotherapy) in early cervical cancer.

Looking into giving chemotherapy on its own before chemo radiotherapy starts for locally advanced cervical cancer testing chemotherapy for advanced cervical cancer.

Radiotherapy

Researchers are looking into ways of improving internal radiotherapy (brachytherapy) for cervical cancer.

They are also looking at increasing the radiation dose when giving external radiotherapy by using Intensity Modulated Radiotherapy (IMRT). The aim is to see if doctors can increase the radiation dose to the cancer, without causing more side effects than standard radiotherapy treatment.

Research is also looking into using different chemotherapy drugs alongside radiotherapy for cervical cancer. Researchers think they might be able to improve results by investigating other combinations of drugs.

Radiotherapy side effects

Researchers for the HOT II trial looked at whether using a high pressure oxygen treatment called hyberbaric oxygen (HBO) therapy could help to relieve the long term side effects of radiotherapy to the area between the hip bones (the pelvis). The results of the trial disagreed with other reports that say HBO is helpful. So the trial team felt larger trials are needed to know for sure.

Another study is looking at using a palm oil supplement and a drug called pentoxifylline to relieve symptoms caused by pelvic radiotherapy. The trial team want to find out if this combination of treatment helps, and to learn more about the side effects.

Researchers are also using a device called an electronic nose to see if they can predict long term changes in bowel function after pelvic radiotherapy.

Targeted cancer drugs

Targeted cancer drugs change the way that cells work. They can boost the body's immune system to fight off or kill cancer cells. Or they can block signals that tell cells to grow.

Research is looking into different types of targeted drugs for cervical cancer. These drugs are being tested in trials. They are being looked at alone or in combination with radiotherapy or chemotherapy to treat cervical cancer.

The drugs being tested include:

Bevacizumab, nivolumab and cediranib

A trial is looking at whether a vaccine against the human papilloma virus (HPV) can work as a treatment against some cancers, including cervical cancer.

Mortality and survival statistics

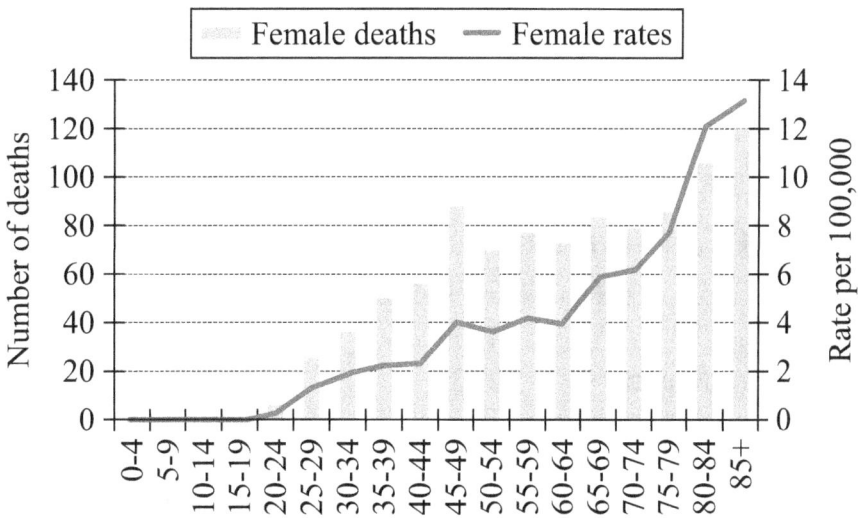

(National Cancer Intelligence Network, 2011).

Figure 5. Number of deaths and age-specific mortality rates for cervical cancer, UK, 2008.

Over 65% of women with cervical cancer survive the disease for five years or more. Survival is higher when diagnosed at a younger age with women under 40 known to have survival rates of about 85%, as seen in Figure 5 above (UKCIS, 2008).

The highest number of deaths occurs in women over 70 who usually do not have regular smear tests anymore.

"Mortality rate is a measure of the number of deaths in general, or due to a specific cause in some population, scaled to the size of that population, per unit time" (Cancer Research, 2011).

In the UK 957 women died from cervical cancer in 2008. This results in a European age-standardised mortality rate of 2.4 per 100,000 females and a basic rate of 3.1 per 100,000 and represents a threefold reduction in death rates over a period of 30 years as can be seen from Table 2 and Figure 6 below.

Table 2. Number of deaths and mortality rates of cervical cancer, UK, 2008 (Modified from UKCIS, 2009).

	England		**Wales**		**Scotland**		**N. Ireland**	
Deaths								
Females	759		68		102		28	
Crude rate per 100,000 population								
Females	2.9		4.4		3.8		3.1	
Age-standardised rate per 100,000 population								
Females	2.3		3.3		2.8		2.5	
95% CI	*2.1*	*2.4*	*2.5*	*4.1*	*2.3*	*3.4*	*1.6*	*3.4*

(UKCIS, 2009)

45

Cervical cancer - survival statistics

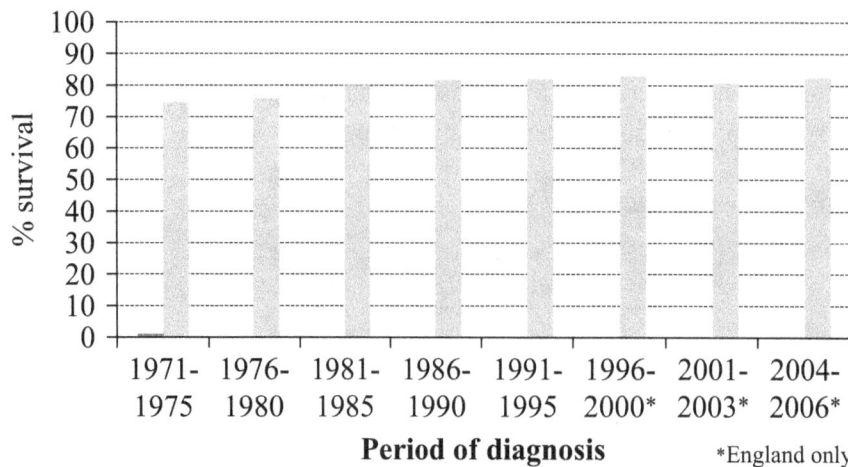

(**National Cancer Intelligence Network, 2011**).

Figure 6. Age-standardised one year relative survival rate, cervical

Cancer, England and Wales 1971–2006

The decrease in cervical cancer mortality is due to increased screening activity across the UK. This decrease is comparable to that achieved across most of Europe although some countries that run less effective screening programmes are witnessing higher mortality rates: countries like Spain, Romania and Bulgaria.

Regular screening translates into early detection, a better prognosis and a high likelihood of curing the disease completely.

DISCUSSION

Lay epidemiology and media representations of cervical cancer in the UK

Lay epidemiology refers to "the processes by which lay people understand and interpret health risks" (Allmark and Tod, 2005 pg 460).

Public Health is impacted negatively when the public does not believe or ignores public health messages. Any good health campaign against cervical cancer should, for example, bring empirical beliefs about the nature of cervical cancer in line with scientific findings and inform about the risks of cervical cancer.

Some current research highlights several empirical beliefs about cervical cancer: that cervical cancer is random, that it is feared and dreaded and that smoking is a well-recognised risk factor (Nielson and Jones, 1998). Hilton and Hunt (2010a) argue that lay knowledge about the main risk factors including HPV is patchy.

This is despite the Department of Health (DoH), spending £3.73 million (over 6% of its annual budget) on advertisements alone promoting the HPV cervical cancer vaccine. This highlights how other information sources and social networks continue to play an important role in forming lay epidemiology.

It is therefore vital to use a better co-ordinated communication strategy. To enable this is however, it is important to understand how cervical cancer has been discussed previously in mainstream media.

Celebrities with cervical cancer

Several celebrities and TV soap personalities have been known to suffer from cervical cancer in the UK in recent years, their experience affecting lay epidemiology significantly.

Top amongst these are Jade Goody and Tanya Jessop from Eastenders. Tanya received her diagnosis following a routine smear test. Jade Goody's story was covered from her diagnosis, through the spreading of her cervical cancer until her death in March 2009 (Hilton and Hunt, 2010a).

It can be argued that though the media attention highlighted the human interest aspects and tragedy of the stories, they represent missed opportunities to educate the public on the risk factors associated with cervical cancer.

How the mass media has reported on cervical cancer in recent years

Mass media (Newspapers, Magazine, Radio, TV etc.) are important in providing information about diseases and prevention methods.

Most newspapers both tabloid and broadsheets tend to provide similar information about early signs and symptoms of cervical cancer although broadsheets are slightly better at discussing risk factors.

Commonly, stories increase popular knowledge about the signs and symptoms but not about the risk factors. Coverage seems to leave out a great deal of information that could mobilise women adequately and does not prioritise the most important threats as understood by public health experts. For example, Radnedge (2011) describes a 13 year old falling into a coma after receiving a dose of the Cervarix vaccine and seems to emphasise the risks of vaccination in a biased way.

Implications

There is still a need to better inform the public about the causes and risk factors of cervical cancers and to explain the public health findings on the benefits of vaccination, cervical screening and lifestyle change suggestions. This can be done in a co-ordinated way, timed to accompany and complement any of the other human interest stories that periodically occur in the mainstream media.

PUBLIC HEALTH SOLUTIONS TO THE CERVICAL CANCER PROBLEM

Currently there is an established multi-faceted strategy to prevent cervical cancer which incorporates the main public health approaches: bio-medical, behavioural or lifestyle and socio-environmental (Laverack, 2004; Sykes, 2007; Wills and Earle, 2007).

The bio-medical approach mainly involves primary prevention by vaccination and secondary prevention by regular cervical screening. Vaccination is the main way of preventing cervical cancer. In September 2008, an HPV immunisation programme was started in the UK targeting schoolgirls with the drug Cervarix from GlaxoSmithKline (GSK). The vaccine targets HPV types 16 and 18 which cause up to 70% of ICCs. Another drug Gardasil which targets these as well as two other strains of HPV responsible for genital warts was not widely accepted, generating controversy in the UK. Earlier introduction of a program of Gardasil could have helped to prevent cases of genital warts as well as ICC, as seen in Australia. The NHS cervical screening programme began in 1988 and has been shown to reduce up to 75% of cervical cancer cases in women in their 50s and 60s who test regularly. Presently, the screening age has been reduced to 12 years from 16, which should yield higher identification rate of HPV infection.

The behavioural approach entails increasing awareness of the causes and risk factors surrounding cervical cancer. This is done on a large scale through leaflets, posters and advertising in mass media which empowers the individual to make healthy choices regarding: diet, smoking, regular exercise and protected sex. It has been argued that over 70% of cervical cancer can be prevented by lifestyle changes alone (Anand et al, 2008). Unfortunately, this approach until now appears mostly expert-led, ignoring input from the individual and sometimes underestimates the encompassing social and physical contexts that predispose or even compel individuals to behave in certain ways. Perhaps refocusing on changing attitudes towards behavioural risk factors would be more effective.

The socio-environmental approach reflects a concerted structural and political approach to fighting cervical cancer in the UK by continuous and persistent lobbying and advocacy for the continuation and expansion of existing policies that wrestle with the wider determinants of health. This involves bigger research budgets, more and better equipped health facilities, day clinics, support lines and addressing inequalities using a community development approach. This approach currently faces the twin hazards of impending budget cuts and changes in political priorities. Besides it is otherwise problematic to exactly specify what a good community means.

Literature review: primary prevention and secondary prevention

- Currently, there is an established multi-faceted strategy to prevent cervical cancer which incorporates the main public health approaches: bio-medical, behavioural or lifestyle and socio-environmental (Laverack, 2004; Sykes, 2007; Wills and Earle, 2007).
- The bio-medical approach mainly involves primary prevention by vaccination and secondary prevention by regular cervical screening.
- Vaccination is the main way of preventing cervical cancer. In September 2008, an HPV immunisation programme was started in the UK targeting schoolgirls with the drug Cervarix from GlaxoSmithKline (GSK).
- The vaccine targets HPV types 16 and 18 which cause up to 70% of ICCs.
- Another drug Gardasil which targets these, as well as two other strains of HPV responsible for genital warts was not widely accepted, generating controversy in the UK.
- Earlier introduction of a Gardasil program could have helped to prevent cases of genital warts as well as ICC, as seen in Australia.
- The NHS cervical screening programme began in 1988 and has been shown to reduce up to 75% of cervical cancer cases in women in their 50s and 60s who test regularly.
- Presently, the screening age has been reduced to 12 years from 16, which should yield a higher identification rate of HPV infection.

Health promotion theories of cervical cancer

Conceptual framework: Behaviour approach

- The behavioural approach entails increasing awareness of the causes and risk factors surrounding cervical cancer.
- A large scale through leaflets, posters and advertising in mass media which empowers the individual to make healthy choices regarding: diet, smoking, regular exercise and protected sex.
- 70% of cervical cancer can be prevented by lifestyle changes alone

- The approach appears mostly expert-led, ignoring input from the individual and underestimates the encompassing social and physical contexts.
- Perhaps refocusing on changing beliefs and attitudes towards behavioural risk factors would be more effective.

Conceptual framework: Socio-environmental approach

- The socio-environmental approach reflects a concerted structural and political approach to fighting cervical cancer in the UK:
- Continuous and persistent lobbying and advocacy for the continuation and expansion of existing policies that wrestle with the wider determinants of health.
- This involves bigger cervical cancer research budgets, more and better equipped health facilities, more day clinics, support lines and addressing inequalities using a community development approach.
- This approach currently faces the twin hazards of impending budget cuts and changes in political priorities. Besides it is otherwise problematic to exactly specify what a good community means.

These preceding solutions address the causations in the epidemiological triangle shown in Figure 3.

Table 3. Cervical Screening Programme results, UK by country, target age-group and target frequency.

	Target age-group	**Frequency of invites**
England	25–64	Every 3 or 5 years
Wales	20–64	Every 3 years
Scotland	20–60	Normal practice
Northern Ireland	20–64	Every 3 or 5 years

Cervical Screening and Vaccination (NHS Cancer Screening Programmes, 2008).

Up to 70% of cervical cancer can be prevented by changes to behaviour (Peto, 1991). This involves mainly improving the lay epidemiology of cervical cancer and the beliefs that support it.

Costs

The main public health costs of cervical cancer are incurred in running both the cervical screening and immunisation programmes. In 2007 this amounted to £157 million pounds (Cancer Research UK, 2011). Additional costs are also incurred in communicating prevention, in research and in developing health facilities.

The main guiding principle on costs is that most individuals in the UK have access to free care on the NHS. They can also choose to use private care but must do so separately, meaning at different times and in different places. This means that individuals can usually not pay extra to receive alternative vaccines for example.

Suggestions of improvements to current strategy for addressing cervical cancer

Currently, the NHS is running a long established public health strategy for combating cervical cancer. This has the advantage that it is has been rolled out UK-wide and health professionals know how it works. Nonetheless, there is room for improvement to the current strategy.

Firstly, it has not been ascertained which method of cervical screening is better: the HPV test or Liquid based cytology (LBC). It is important to carry out randomised trials to establish which one is more effective (simple, less errors, cost efficient) and then roll it out NHS-wide. Ways of improving the current coverage of cervical cancer screening from 78.9% in 2008/9 can be investigated (NHS Cancer Screening Programme, 2011).

Secondly, alternative vaccines to Cervarix for cervical cancer are available. It is important to revisit the procurement issue and consider substitutes to Cervarix, which is the chosen vaccine on the NHS programme. Gardasil, for example, which provides the added benefit over Cervarix of protecting against two extra strains of HPV which cause anogenital warts could represent better value for money.

Improvement on international co-operation would represent an added bonus to the cervical cancer prevention agenda. There is strong evidence that the UK could learn from other European countries like Malta, Switzerland and Finland which have lower incidence and mortality rates despite spending comparatively less on cervical cancer prevention (ECCA, 2009).

More can also be done to improve behaviour counselling provided by the NHS. This can be done by offering more clinics, but more importantly by embedding cervical cancer prevention in other campaigns (Such as the fight against obesity or STDs) so that there is a more holistic approach to tackling the disease.

CONCLUSION

This report examines the epidemiology of cervical cancer in the UK. Using epidemiological data from multiple sources, it finds that there is still a gap between the lay epidemiology for the disease and desired public health expert outcomes. This means that despite advances in cervical cancer research outlined herein, the disease remains a threat and the current strategy can be improved further. In the light of impending budget cuts, more has to be done to improve the cost versus benefit ratio and some alterations to the current strategy are made.

REFERENCES

Allmark, P and Tod, A. (2006). How should public health professionals engage with lay epidemiology? Journal of Medical Ethics. 32 (10), P460–463.

Anand, P., Kunnumakara, A.B., Sundaram, C., Harikumar, K.B, Tharakan, S.T., Lai, O.S., Sung, B. and Aggarwal, B.B. (2008). Cancer is a Preventable Disease that Requires Major Lifestyle Changes. Pharmaceutical Research. 25 (9), P2097–2116.

Ault, K.A. (2007). Human papillomavirus vaccines and the potential for cross-protection between related HPV types. Gynaecologic Oncology. 107 (Issue 2, Supplement), s31–s33.

Barker, D.J.P. and Rose, G. (1984) Epidemiology in medical practice, 3rd Edition, Edinburgh: Churchill Livingstone.

Bell, L., and Seale, C. (2010). The reporting of cervical cancer in the mass media: a study of UK newspapers. European Journal of Cancer Care. 20 (1), P389–394.

Bosch, F. X., Lorincz, A., Muñoz, N., M Meijer, C. J. L., and Shah, K.V. (2002). The causal relation between human papillomavirus and cervical cancer. Journal of Clinical Pathology. 55 (1), P244–265.

Cancer Research UK. (2011). Cervical cancer statistics-UK. Available: http://info.cancerresearchuk. org/cancerstats/types/cervix/?script=true. Last accessed 01st Dec 2010.

Clifford, G.M, Smith, J.S., Aguado, T., and Franceschi, S. (2003). Comparison of HPV type distribution in high-grade cervical lesions and cervical cancer: a meta-analysis. British Journal of Cancer. 89 (1), P101–105.

Comber, H., and Gavin, A. (2004). Recent trends in cervical cancer mortality in Britain and Ireland: the case for population-based cervical cancer screening. British Journal of Cancer. 91 (1), P1902–1904.

Cuzick, J, Castanon, A., and Sasieni, P. (2010). Predicted impact of vaccination against human papillomavirus 16/18 on cancer incidence and cervical abnormalities in women aged 20–29 in the UK. British Journal of Cancer. 102 (5), P933–939.

ECCA. (2011). HPV Vaccination across Europe. Available: http://www.ecca.info/fileadmin/user_upload/HPV_Vaccination/ECCA_HPV_Vaccination_April_2009.pdf. Last accessed 01 Dec 2011.

Everett, T., Bryant, A., Griffin, M.F., Martin-Hirsch, P.P.L., Forbes, C.A., and Jepson, R.G. (2011). Interventions targeted at women to encourage the uptake of cervical screening (Review). The Cochrane Collaboration. 21 (5), P1–94.

Franceschi S. The IARC commitment to cancer prevention: The example of papillomavirus and cervical cancer. Recent Results in Cancer Research 2005; 166:277–297.

Gordis, L (1996). Epidemiology. Philadelphia Pennsylvania: W.B Saunders Company. P31–32.

Grainge, M.J., Seth, R., Coupland, C., Guo, L., Rittman, T., Vryenhoef, P., Johnson. Jenkins, D., and Neal, K.R. (2005). Human papillomavirus infection in women who develop high-grade cervical intraepithelial neoplasia or cervical cancer: a case–control study in the UK. British Journal of Cancer. 92 (1), P1794–1799.

Green, J., Gonzalez, A.B., Sweetland, S., Beral, V., Chilvers, C., Crossley, B., Deacon, J., Hermon, C., Jha, P., Mant, D., Peto, J., Pike, M., and Vessey, M.P. (2003). Risk factors for adenocarcinoma and squamous cell carcinoma of the cervix in women aged 20–44 years: the UK National Case–Control Study of Cervical Cancer. British Journal of Cancer. 89 (11), P2078–2086.

Henderson, L., Clements, A., Damery, S., Wilkinson, C., Austoker, J., and Wilson, S. (2011). 'A false sense of security'? Understanding the role of the HPV vaccine on future cervical screening behaviour: a qualitative study of UK parents and girls of vaccination age. Journal of Medical Screening. 18 (1), P41–45.

Hilton, S and Hunt, K. (2010). Coverage of Jade Goody's cervical cancer in UK newspapers: a missed opportunity for health promotion? Journal of BioMed Central Public Health. 368 (10), P1–8.

Hilton, S., Hunt, K., Langan, M., Bedford, H., and Petticrew, M. (2010). Newsprint media representations of the introduction of the HPV vaccination programme for cervical cancer prevention in the UK (2005–2008). Journal of Social Science and Medicine. 70 (1), P942–950.

Johnson, C.S and Philip, Z. (2004). An evaluation of liquid-based cytology and human papillomavirus. British Journal of Cancer. 91 (1), P84–91.

Kemohan, E.E.M. (1996). Evaluation of a pilot study for breast and cervical cancer screening with Bradford's minority ethnic women; a community development approach, 1991–93. British Journal of Cancer. 74 (1), P42–46.

Kohli, M., Ferko, N., Martin, A., Franco, E.L., Jenkins, D., Gallivan, S., Johnson, C.S., and Drummond, M. (2007). Estimating the long-term impact of a prophylactic human papillomavirus 16/18 vaccine on the burden of cervical cancer in the UK. British Journal of Cancer. 96 (1), P143–150.

Kulasingam, S.L., Benard, S., Barnabas, R.V., Largeron, N., and Myers, E.R. (2008). Adding aquadrivalent human papillomavirus vaccine to the UK cervical cancer screening programme: A cost-effectiveness analysis. Journal of BioMed Central: Cost Effectiveness and Resource. 6 (4), P1–11.

Lewison, G., Tootell, S., Roe, P., and Sullivan, R. (2008). How do the media report cancer research? A study of the UK's BBC website. British Journal of Cancer. 99 (1), P569–576.

Marmot, M (2005) Social determinants of health inequalities. Lancet 365 (19): 1099–104.

Martin-Hirsch, P.L. (2011). Cervical cancer (updated). International Journal of Cancer. 128 (1), P927–935.

Moreno V, Bosch FX, Munoz N, et al. Effect of oral contraceptives on risk of cervical cancer in women with human papillomavirus infection: The IARC multicentric case-control study. Lancet 2002; 359(9312):1085–1092.

Munoz, N., Bosch, X. F., Sanjose, S., Herrero, R., Castellsague, X., Shah, K.V., Snijders, P.J.F., and Meijer, J.L.M. (2003). Epidemiologic Classification of Human Papillomavirus Types Associated with Cervical Cancer. The New England Journal of Medicine. 348 (6), P518–527.

Nair, M. S., Bhandari, H. M. and Nordin, A. J. (2007). Cervical cancer in women aged less than 25: East Kent experience. Journal of Obstetrics and Gynaecology. 27 (7), P706–708.

National Cancer Intelligence Network. (2011). Profile of Cervical Cancer in England Incidence, Mortality and Survival. Available: www.ncin.org.uk/view.aspx?rid=496. Last accessed 01st Dec 2011.

Neilson, A., Jones, K.R., and FColl, F. (1998). Women's lay knowledge of cervical cancer/cervical screening: accounting for non-attendance at cervical screening clinics. Journal of advanced Nursing. 28 (3), P571–575.

NHS. (2011). About Cervical Screening. Available: http://cancerscreening.nhs.uk/cervical/about-cervical-screening.html. Last accessed 01st Dec 2011.

Office of National Statistics. (2011). Topic guide to: Conditions and Diseases. Available: http://www.statistics.gov.uk/hub/health-social-care/health-of-the-population/conditions-and-diseases. Last accessed 01st Dec 2011.

Powell, N.G., Hibbitts, S.J., Boyde, A.M., Newcombe, R.G., Tristram, A.J., and Fiander, A.N. (2011). The risk of cervical cancer associated with specific types of human papillomavirus: a case–control study in a UK population. International Journal of Cancer. 128 (1), P1676–1682.

Radnedge, A. (2011) Cervical cancer jab leaves girl aged 13 in a 'waking coma.' METRO, 15 November, p.5.

Salz, T., Gottlieb, S.L, Smith, J.S., and Brewer, N.T. (2010). The Association between Cervical Abnormalities and Attitudes Toward Cervical Cancer Prevention. Journal of Women's Health. 19 (11), P2011–2016.

Sasieni, P., Adams, J., and Cuzick, J. (2003). Benefit of cervical screening at different ages: evidence from the UK audit of screening histories. British Journal of Cancer. 89 (1), P88–93.

Schnatz, P.F., Markelova, N.V., Holmes, D., Mandavilli, S.R., and O'sullivan, D.M. (2008). The Prevalence of Cervical HPV and Cytological Abnormalities in Association with Reproductive: Factors of Rural Nigerian Women. Journal of Women's Health. 17 (2), P279–285.

Smith JS, Green J, Berrington de GA, et al. Cervical cancer and use of hormonal contraceptives: A systematic review. Lancet 2003; 361 (9364):1159–1167.

Smith, J.S., Green, J., Gonzalez, A.B., Appleby, P., Peto, J., Plummer, M., Franceschi, S., and Beral, V. (2003). Cervical cancer and use of hormonal contraceptives: a systematic review. The Journal of Lancet. 361 (1), P1159–1167.

4

THE EPIDEMIOLOGY OF END OF LIFE GLOBALLY USING OF MORPHINE

Johnson Mbabazi and Mohammed Sattar

ABSTRACT

The book explains the importance of both palliative and end of life care in both developing and developed countries. It uses Pakistan and Uganda as examples on how to improve palliative care particularly in managing pain symptoms using morphine as a drug to ensure comfort in patients and reducing stress to patient relatives. It also underlines ethical considerations that needs to be addressed in providing treatment particularly in cancer patients. This helps in reducing stress and finding best way forward in providing treatment with chronic conditions as well as managing the condition better. Cancer: Palliative Care and end of life conditions examines the nature of the care and support that can be provided to those in need of palliative care and their families. This covers not only the physical treatment, such as pain management, but also the psychological well-being of patients. Health workers, clinicians, specialist nurses, general practitioners, hospital doctors and medical students will find a balanced and considerate overview of the subject which will be of value in managing patients and helping them to come to terms with their condition. Lastly this book is a clinical guidelines, and advice on controlling symptoms, as well as showing doctors and carers how to provide physical and psychological comfort. It helps the clinician to develop a scientific approach to managing symptoms. In the United Kingdom ampoules of morphine is destroyed in the name of health and safety yet in developing counties such as Zimbabwe people are dying agonising death

INTRODUCTION

The epidemiology of end of life globally

The published statistics will be used on a range of health and long-term conditions to inform debate, decision-making and research both within different global government the wider communities worldwide to help improve palliative care in managing symptoms and improving clinical care in order hospitals, hospices, nursing homes, residential homes and those acquiring care from homes with the help of general practitioners.

The term 'palliative care' can be defined as the treatment, care and support for people with a life-limiting illness, and their family and friends. It's sometimes called 'supportive care'.

The aim of palliative care is to help patients or clients have a good quality of life. This includes being as well and active as possible in the time patients have left. It can involve:

- Social care, including help with things like washing, dressing or eating
- Support for your family and friends
- Managing physical symptoms such as pain
- Emotional, spiritual and psychological support

Palliative care

Palliative care is given to patients with a life limiting illness. This is an illness that can't be cured and that patients or clients are more likely to die from. You could hear this type of illness called 'life-threatening' or 'terminal'. People might also use the terms 'progressive' (gets worse over time) or 'advanced' (is at a serious stage) to describe these illnesses. Examples of life-limiting illnesses include advanced cancer, motor neuron disease (MND) and dementia.

Patients could receive palliative care at any stage in their illness. Having palliative care doesn't necessarily mean that a patient is likely to die soon. Some people receive palliative care for years. Patients could also have palliative care alongside treatments, therapies and medicines aimed at controlling their illness, such as chemotherapy or radiotherapy. However, palliative care does include caring for people who are nearing the end of life.

End of life care

End of life care involves treatment, care and support for individuals who are nearing the end of their life. It's an important part of palliative care. It is for individuals who are thought to be in the last year of life, but this timeframe can be difficult to predict. Some people might only receive end of life care in their last weeks or days.

End of life care aims to help people to live as comfortably as possible in the time one may have left. It involves managing physical symptoms and getting emotional support for the patient and his or her family and friends. Patients might require more of this type of care towards the end of your life.

End of life care also involves talking to patients and their family and friends about what to expect towards the end of their lives. The family members or relatives looking after patients on end of life will talk to patients about their needs and wishes, and make sure they consider what their patients want in the care they provide.

HOW DO I GET PALLIATIVE OR END OF LIFE CARE?

DEVELOPED COUNTRIES FOR EXAMPLE UNITED KINGDOM

For people living in developed countries speak to your General practitioners (family doctors) or another healthcare professional about how palliative or end of life care might help you and how you can access it.

If you are a family member or friend of the person who is ill, you may be able to access support for yourself. If the person who is ill is receiving care from a hospice or other local service, you may also be able to get support from them. Even if the person who's ill doesn't want to have palliative or end of life care, you can still get support.

INITIATING PALLIATIVE CARE IN DEVELOPING COUNTRIES

Developing counties (low or middle income country) For example; Uganda, Pakistan and many others. It is estimated that more than one billion people (85% of world population) live in the developing countries with 20% global gross resources only. Thus, most of the developing countries remain grossly insufficient in their respective healthcare system. Ever since the independence of each developing country, many government nations are struggling to develop healthcare systems. During the last two decades, a quick progress has been witnessed in this field, but it largely remained limited to private sector health institutions, with limited progress made by public sector. Yet palliative care (PC) remained a highly neglected area and even big academic institutions, private or government, have no PC services or programs.

JUSTIFICATION FOR NEED OF PALLIATIVE CARE

The justification for the need of palliative care is that; supportive care helps the patient and their family to cope with their condition and treatment of it from pre-diagnosis, through the process of diagnosis and treatment, to cure, continuing illness or death and into bereavement. It helps the patient to maximise the benefits of treatment and to live as well as possible with the effects of the disease. It is given equal priority alongside diagnosis and treatment. Palliative care is part of supportive care. It holds several elements of supportive care. It has been defined by The National Institute for Health and Care Excellence (NICE) as: Palliative care is the active holistic care of patients with advanced progressive illness. Management of pain and other symptoms and provision of psychological, social and spiritual support is paramount. The goal of palliative care is achievement of the best quality of life for patients and their families.

Several aspects of PC are also applicable earlier in the course of the illness in conjunction with other treatments. PC is an emerging medical specialty which enhances the patient's overall quality of life by providing a wide range of services. In current modern practice the concept of PC has been changed. It does not mean the end of life care for dying patient only, but rather it is an approach that improves quality of life for patients suffering from incurable chronic and life threatening illness and to provide support for patient's families.

WHO PROVIDES PALLIATIVE CARE?

The professionals involved in your care will depend on what sort of care and support you need. Palliative care can be provided in different places including in your home, in hospital, in a care home or nursing home, and in a hospice.

GENERAL CARE PROFESSIONALS

General health and social care professionals give day to day palliative care to people as part of their roles. Patients might see these people regularly as part of their care:

- social workers
- care workers

- Spiritual care professionals
- Family doctors (GPs)
- district or community nurses

These professionals should be involved as early as possible after patients have been diagnosed. They will assess patients' needs and wishes, and those of patients' families and friends. They might refer patients to specialist care if patients need it.

SPECIALIST CARE PROFESSIONALS

Specialist palliative care professionals are experts in providing palliative care and will have training and experience in this area. They might be involved in managing more complex care problems. Specialists usually work in teams to provide joined-up care and patients might see one or more specialists if they are referred to them.

Specialist teams include:

- palliative care doctors
- nurse specialists (Respiratory nurses for emphysema or bronchitis patients, diabetic nurse for diabetic nurse or palliative team for palliative patients)
- Specialist health professionals, such as physiotherapists, occupational therapists, dieticians and social workers. Specialist palliative care services may be provided by the NHS (Health and Social Care in Northern Ireland), local councils or voluntary organisations.
- Counsellors

Palliative care, while still a relatively new element to modern healthcare, is increasingly recognised as an essential part of all healthcare systems. Despite this, it is broadly acknowledged that there is still insufficient access to hospice and palliative care worldwide, and with an ageing population who are going to be living and dying with more complex conditions such as cancer, AIDS, Diabetes, heart failure, angina, stroke, dementia, Parkinson disease, the demand for care is only going to increase.

The need for palliative care has never been greater and is increasing at a rapid pace due to the world's ageing population and increases in cancer and other non-communicable diseases. Despite this need, palliative care is underdeveloped in most of the world, and outside North America, Europe, and Australia, access to quality palliative care is very rare.

PAKISTAN AS A DEVELOPING COUNTRY

Pakistan is a developing country of South East Asia, with all the incumbent difficulties currently being faced by the region. Insufficient public healthcare facilities, poorly regulated private health sector, low budgetary allocation for health, improper priority setting while allocating limited resources, have resulted essentially in an absence of palliative care from the healthcare scene. Almost 90% of healthcare expenditure is out of the patient's pocket with more than 45% of population living below the poverty line. All these factors have a collective potential to translate into an end of life care disaster as a large percentage of population is suffering from chronic debilitating or terminal diseases. So far, such a disaster has not materialised, the reason being a family based culture emphasising the care of the sick and old at home, supported by religious teachings.

This culture is not limited to Pakistan but subsists in the entire sub-continent, where looking after the sick/elderly at home is considered to be the duty of the younger generation. With effects of globalisation, more and older people are living alone and an increasing need for palliative care is being realised. However, there does not seem to be any plan on the part of the public or private sectors to initiate palliative care services.

This book seeks to trace the social and cultural perspectives in developing and developed counties with regards to accessing palliative care in the context of healthcare facilities available, why morphine must be provided in cancer patients to control symptoms in developing counties such as Uganda and Pakistan.

PALLIATIVE CARE IN UGANDA

Palliative care was first introduced to Uganda in 1993 with the start of Hospice Uganda (HU). At that time, there was already supportive care for HIV/AIDS patients with home care from TASO (the AIDS Support organization) and many other home care programs. These organizations supported "clients" and their families with mainly counselling; they encouraged living positively with HIV. TASO in particular made a huge impact on attitudes to HIV/AIDS in the country and to education towards prevention of the disease. This is now having positive effects, with a reduction in the infection rates among pregnant women in several centres in the country.

Recently, palliative care has been attracting funds. Like many other countries, Uganda's AIDS support organizations are now described as having palliative care, yet they do not have the modern methods of pain and symptom control introduced through the modern hospice movement by Dame Cicely Saunders, and researched since 1967. Nurses are the backbone of palliative care. The emphasis on counselling by donor agencies, with provision of salaries higher than for nurses, has taken nurses from their profession to become counsellors. Counsellors are frustrated when faced with a patient in severe pain and neither the patient nor family can be counselled due to their distress from the pain.

Uganda is now trying to address this problem and the great need for palliative care in HIV/AIDS and/ or cancer by grafting pain and symptom control onto already existing support organizations. Palliative care is also being introduced throughout the existing health systems in the country, with support from the Ministry of Health, using HU as their technical experts. Palliative care is now part of essential clinical services for HIV/AIDS patients in the five-year Strategic health Plan from 2000 to 2005.

GOVERNMENT GIVE LOW PRIORITY TO PALLIATIVE CARE IN DEVELOPING COUNTIES

In many resource poor countries, death is accompanied by avoidable pain and other distressing symptoms. Unfortunately, governments in these countries usually give care at the end of life a low priority compared with preventive and curative services. This prioritisation makes little sense, especially when applied to treating patients with cancer and HIV (Human Immune Virus) or AIDS (Acquired Immune Deficiency Syndrome), since prevention efforts are often failing to reduce the disease burden, while treatments aimed at cure or prolonging life are still too expensive to be made widely available.

As a few physicians in Uganda, Jamaica and Rwanda, believe that providing quality care at the end of life should be seen as a global public health priority. By using relatively low-cost palliative care approaches and community-based strategies, thousands of terminally ill patients in Africa and the Caribbean could be relieved of their pain and suffering.

Palliative care is expanding in the developed world in spite of myths and misunderstanding about its nature and purpose, but is only beginning to be available in the developing world where it is needed most.

Since the early 1980s, the need for palliative care for cancer patients has been progressively acknowledged worldwide. More recently, there is increased awareness of the need for palliative care for other chronic diseases or conditions such as HIV/AIDS, congestive heart failure, cerebrovascular disease, neurodegenerative disorders, chronic respiratory diseases, drug-resistant tuberculosis, and diseases of older people. However, there remains a huge unmet need for palliative care for these chronic life-limiting health problems in most parts of the world.

PALLIATIVE CARE IN PAKISTAN

In a study of Asia Pacific Hospice Palliative Care Network (APHN), written by Fr. Robert McCulloch, Home-Based Palliative Nursing at St. Elizabeth Hospital, Hyderabad, Pakistan explains the difficulties in Pakistan terminally-ill patients are treated as sources of income by the medical profession and the hospital culture. Their illness is not relieved and the financial situation of their families is wrecked as they seek for a cure or for pain relief. This is not unethical for patients and their families that seek for comfort who are on end of life or palliative.

It is even concerning that Pakistan government and hospitals are not considering ethical consideration of managing patient symptoms as the Palliative Care Department at St. Elizabeth Hospital depends on donations. The Melbourne Overseas Mission of the archdiocese of Melbourne helped to purchase a small car to enable the palliative care nurses to visit patients. Some of the equipment such as syringe drivers for continuous pain-killing medication is expensive. The families of patients have little, there is no insurance cover, and the government gives nothing. This means that patients with no money remain untreated and die quicker. This leads to high mortality rate and early death in human life. This is unethical as well.

Epidemiology of pain in cancer and/or AIDS

The estimated population of Uganda is now 22 million. The incidence of HIV/AIDS has decreased from 30% in the early 1990's to 6% of the population in 2002. This reduction is considered to be due to a number of factors:

- The acknowledgment of the disease in Uganda by President Museveni early on in the epidemic, bringing in aid for VCT and prevention.
- The publicity given in schools and in the media to the use of prevention and abstinence.
- Special programs through Churches "Youth Alive" involving youth in supporting each other in abstinence.
- The positive attitude towards HIV/AIDS due to organizations, such as TASO (The AIDS support Organization), which have encouraged people to be open about their status and to advise others in their age cohort and communities on how to avoid the disease.
- However, the epidemic of death is still with us. The infective rate is down but many are still dying

of HIV/AIDS and related cancers. It was estimated that 0.1% of the population were suffering from cancer before the onset of the HIV epidemic.

- Overall, 40–60% of all cancers attending hospice and registered with the Cancer Registry of Uganda are HIV-related, so this estimate is probably now too low. Using 0.1%, it is estimated that there are 22,000 new cancer cases each year. Twenty-five percent of cancers presenting to HU are epidemic Kaposi's sarcoma. A further 25% are estimated to be HIV-associated, from the course of the disease. This in itself brings up the incidence of cancer countrywide.

- All patients with cancer attending HU are in pain. One percent of the population is suffering at any one time from AIDS pain. This gives us an estimate that 240,000 are presently in pain in Uganda on a daily basis.

- However, when looking at pain and symptom control, pain is compounded in the patient suffering from Stage 4 AIDS and cancer. Although pain in AIDS may be temporary if the opportunistic infection is controlled, pain recurs and needs constant monitoring. The commonest severe pains seen at HU in HIV/AIDS are cryptococcal meningitis, esophageal ulceration, herpes simplex, herpes zoster, and peripheral neuropathies.

CONTROLLING PAIN SYMPTOMS USING MORPHINE IN CANCER PATIENTS STAGE 4

It is unfortunate in some hospitals in Uganda (Nsabya hospital) for stage 4 cancer patients are being given morphine just weeks if at all they give it before they die despite 'enduring intense pain for months. Doctors are waiting too long before giving patients with advanced cancer pain relief, new research suggests.

Terminally ill patients are often not prescribed powerful opioid painkillers, such as morphine, until just nine weeks before their death, a study found. Although Mulago Cancer Institute (Uganda) gives morphine but this emotionally traumatic to patients and their families seeing patients go through such pain.

I also believe it is unethical only following an intended operation because is what was diagnosed in private hospitals yet a patient could be developing and metastasising cancer at rapid rate yet if seen early responding to treatment is better. The diagnosis and management of cancer is so poor in Uganda yet it is increasing at a faster rate as a silent killer.

I also believe it is unethical to only provide treatment following an early diagnosis for cancer patients globally if patients do not have money or medical insurance must not be treated. Medicine and health care is aimed at preservation of life, management of long-term illness, promoting palliative care to provide fulfilling patient care and ensuring end of care services are satisfactory to patients and their families globally. This is humanity and humility should countries respond to this as all people pay taxes worldwide in their respective countries. Even if it is end of life let people die with dignity, satisfied care and fulfilment. Otherwise, many of them will have been suffering pain over a much longer period of time.

Clinical advantages and disadvantages of using morphine in cancer patients

- Among the benefits of taking morphine for cancer is the relief of pain and the comfort of the patient's family and friends who are concerned about their loved one's pain control.
- The negative aspects of taking morphine for cancer include various adverse side effects, such as chronic constipation. The acceleration of the growth of cancer cells and their spread throughout the body are perhaps the most serious drawbacks of morphine for cancer.

- Giving morphine for cancer pain relief is relatively common in palliative care because it provides comfort for many terminally ill patients who might otherwise spend their final days in discomfort.
- Using this drug not only helps the patient rest, his or her family members and friends also are indirectly comforted knowing that their loved one's suffering is being controlled.
- Some patients hold strong convictions against taking a narcotic even for medicinal purposes, and the existence of such beliefs could be considered one of the cons of using morphine for cancer.
- Pain relief for the patient and some sense of comfort for his or her family and friends, however, probably are the only two pros of using morphine for cancer.
- Overall if morphine is provided with correct dose depending on the kevels pain and wishes of patient must be provided to reduce pain symptoms as opposed to hospital policies particularly in developing countries.

ADVICE ON CANCER PAIN

Pain is usually a sign that something is wrong. It is a sign that an individual has an illness or an injury. When there is damage to any part of a person's body, nervous system sends a message along nerves to his or her brain. When the brain receives these messages, the individual feel pain. This includes pain caused by cancer.

Having a lot of pain can be terrifying. It can make patients and their families think that cancer must be growing. But how much pain a patient has is not necessarily connected to a cancer's growth. A very small tumour that's pressing on a nerve or a patient's spinal cord can be extremely painful. Yet a very large tumour somewhere else might not cause a patient any pain at all.

Having pain after successful treatment doesn't necessarily mean that cancer has come back. Some people get pain after cancer treatments like surgery or radiotherapy. It might be a long term side effect of chemotherapy.

Post-treatment pain like this can start or get worse months or even years after treatment. It's due to the nervous system rewiring itself after damage to the nerves. The nerves then send pain signals.

Often, this type of pain doesn't respond to ordinary painkillers. Patient cancer specialist will then use other ways of treating pain. This includes using other medicines. Remember that pain might not be related to patient's cancer. It's completely understandable to worry about this. But sometimes pain can just be due to everyday things like arthritis, headaches, constipation or digestive problems.

NOT ALL CANCERS CAUSE PAIN

Many people with cancer do not have pain. This is because cancers don't have any nerves of their own. The pain comes from a tumour pressing on nerves nearby.

Between 3 and 6 out of 10 people with cancer (30 to 60%) have some sort of pain. With advanced cancer, pain is more likely. Advanced cancer means the cancer has spread or come back since it was first treated. Some studies have shown up to 9 out of 10 people with advanced cancer (up to 90%) have pain. It is possible to relieve all pain to some extent with the right treatment. With good pain control, most people should be able to be free of pain when they are lying down or sitting.

The best way of controlling pain depends on what's causing it. The first step is to tell a general practitioner in developed countries and in developing countries go check it out in hospitals by a doctor.

HOW PAIN AFFECTS AN INDIVIDUAL

Pain can affect a person physically and emotionally. It is a very personal experience that feels different to everyone. What is painful and disturbing for one person might not affect someone else so much. Everyone needs different pain treatment. What works for one patient might not necessarily help someone else. So having an individual treatment plan to control for pain is very important.

Lastly, general practitioners always advise clients to always try to write down as much detail as possible about their individual pain, including when it comes on and what it feels like. This will help cancer specialist if diagnosed with cancer to find out what's causing it and the best way of treating it.

For example; things to write down on a piece of paper or an email include;

What it feels like – for example, stabbing, aching or burning
Where it is – in one place, or spread around an area
What relieves it – for example, heat, cold, changing position, massage
How often you have it – always or it comes and goes
How it comes on - suddenly or gradually.

UNDERSTANDING PAINKILLERS

There are several different types and strengths of painkiller. It's important to get the right type and to take them regularly, as prescribed by your doctor or pharmacist advises you to. These must be registered pharmacists and registered doctors.

Painkillers are also called analgesics or analgesia. The type you have depends on the kind of pain you have.

- For mild pain, you usually have simple painkillers, such as paracetamol
- For moderate pain, you usually have treatment with opioid painkillers, such as codeine
- For ongoing or severe pain, you usually have morphine type opioid painkillers

Patients might also take other types of drugs alongside the painkillers, depending on the pain. These include:

- anti-inflammatory drugs such as ibuprofen (Nurofen)
- anti-depressants or anti-epileptic drugs (nerve pain)

An experienced doctor can judge which type of painkiller is best for their patient. The important thing is that patients have the right type for their individual pain and the right dose.

EXAMPLES OF STUDIES THAT DEMONSTRATE ORAL MORPHINE MANAGES PAIN IN CANCER PATIENTS

Oral morphine for cancer pain

Research study from Cochrane systematic review by McQuay H, 2019 demonstrated that oral Morphine (taken by mouth) is an effective pain-killer for cancer pain. Pain is commonly experienced by people with cancer, and morphine is considered the gold standard for relieving pain when it becomes moderate to severe. This review aimed to assess the effectiveness of oral morphine, and 54 studies were found. However, the majority of these studies were designed to show that different formulations of morphine were effective, and this made it difficult to extract useful information on the effectiveness of morphine itself. Nevertheless, these trials show that morphine gives good relief for cancer pain but with some unwanted effects, mainly constipation and nausea and vomiting.

Ketamine as an adjuvant to opioids for cancer pain

Research study from Cochrane systematic review by Bell R.F, Eccleston, C, Kalso EA. Cochrane Database of Systematic Reviews 2018, showed the benefits and harms of adding ketamine to strong pain-killers such as morphine for the relief of cancer pain are not yet established. Morphine-like drugs (opioids) are frequently prescribed for moderate and severe cancer pain, but in some cases these drugs are not effective. Ketamine, an anaesthetic agent, is used to improve analgesia when opioids alone are ineffective. However, evidence for the effectiveness of this practice is limited. Two small studies suggest that when ketamine is given with morphine it may help to control cancer pain. However, these data are insufficient to assess the effectiveness of ketamine in this setting.

Celiac plexus block for pancreatic cancer pain in adults

Research study from Cochrane systematic review by Arcidiacono PG, Calori G, Carrara S, McNicol ED, Testoni PA. Cochrane Database of Systematic Reviews 2018 have proved that abdominal pain is a major symptom in patients with inoperable pancreatic cancer and is often difficult to treat. Celiac plexus block (CPB) is a safe and effective method for reducing this pain. It involves the chemical destruction of the nerve fibres that convey pain from the abdomen to the brain. We searched for studies comparing CPB with standard analgesic therapy in patients with inoperable pancreatic cancer. We were interested in the primary outcome of pain, measured on a visual analogue scale (VAS). We also looked at the amount of opioid (morphine-like drugs) patients took (opioid consumption) and adverse effects of the treatment. Six studies (358 participants) comparing CPB with standard therapy (painkillers) met our inclusion criteria. At four weeks pain scores were significantly lower in the CPB group. Opioid consumption was also significantly lower than in the control group. The main adverse effects were diarrhoea or constipation (this symptom was significantly more likely in the control group, where opioid consumption was higher). Endoscopic ultrasonography (EUS)-guided CPB is becoming popular as a minimally invasive technique that has fewer risks, but we were not able to find any RCTs assessing this method (current medical literature on this subject is limited to studies without control groups). Although the data on EUS-guided CPB and pain control are promising, we await rigorously designed RCTs that may validate these findings. We conclude that, although statistical evidence is minimal for the superiority of pain relief over analgesic therapy, the fact that CPB causes fewer adverse effects than opioids is important for patients.

CONCLUSION

Morphine is effective and satisfactory in managing pain symptoms in cancer patients as studies have demonstrated. Both palliative and end of life care in both developing and developed countries all need to practice right ethical considerations in managing pain symptoms in cancer patients according to the patient's wish. This has been poor in developing countries such as Pakistan and Uganda. There is a need to improve palliative care particularly in managing pain symptoms using morphine as a drug to ensure comfort in patients and reducing stress to patient relatives. It also underlines ethical considerations that needs to be addressed in providing treatment particularly in cancer patients. This helps in reducing stress and finding best way forward in providing treatment with chronic conditions as well as managing the condition better. In the United Kingdom ampoules of morphine is destroyed in the name of health and safety yet in developing counties such as Zimbabwe people are dying agonising death.

ACKNOWLEDGEMENT AND DEDICATION

I want to acknowledge Dr. Mohammed Sattar a general practitioner in England who emphasised in writing this research and an author of this research, my late Father Mr. Fred Luwaga who died malignant neoplasm of the liver and intrapatic bile ducts (pancreatic cancer) and requested me to write a book on cancer following our long trip to Ekimega –Uganda to grave sites where we were paying our tribute to our lost loved ones little did I know he was saying good bye. More importantly asked to write a book to help others. I dedicate this book to you Father Mr. Luwaga Fred your legacy will always stand and stays beyond a tombstone or a graveyard I love you so much always. We want also want to dedicate all those people and families who are on end of life care, palliative care and doctors globally in both developing countries (Uganda and Pakistan) and developed countries all around the world. We know it will help you manage, make right choices and better decision making in long-term illness for example cancer, diabetes, cardiovascular diseases, dementia during palliative or end of life care.

5

THE BOOK OF GLOBAL UNDERSTANDING OF HIV AND AIDS

Johnson Mbabazi

ABSTRACT

There are about 34.7 million people worldwide living with HIV/AIDS. Half are women. There has been an affected global increase in the rates of women living with HIV/AIDS. Among young women, especially in developing countries, infection rates are rapidly increasing. This book is going to focus on Uganda as an example of a developing country and our Preventative International Care (Non-governmental organisation). Preventative care international (PCI) is NGO (Non-governmental Organisation) founded in 2013. Aims at preventing HIV in women, children and adult men. The PCI Organisation aimed at preventing HIV in women, children and adult men, to have a free community that is free from HIV/AIDS and reproductive health challenges and to sensitise both rural and urban areas on dangers of STIs, HIV and AIDS.

Many of these women are also mothers with children. When a woman is labelled, stereotyped as having HIV, she is treated with suspicion and her morality is being questioned. Current research has suggested that women living with HIV/AIDS can be affected by delay in diagnosis, inferior access to health care services, internalised stigma and a poor utilisation of health services. This makes it extremely difficult for women to take care of their own health needs. Women are also reluctant to disclose their HIV-positive status as they fear this may result in physical feelings of shame, social exclusion, violence, or expulsion from home. Women living with HIV/AIDS who are also mothers carry a particularly heavy burden of being HIV-infected.

This book can be used as evidence for health care providers to implement socially and culturally appropriate services to assist individuals and groups who are living with HIV/AIDS in many societies. The book is of interest to infected individuals, scholars and students, social work, nursing, public health and medicine and health professionals who have a specific interest in issues concerning women who are mothers and living with HIV/AIDS from cross-cultural perspective.

ABBREVIATIONS IN FULL

Preventive Care International (PCI)

Uganda Fish Processors & Exporters Association (UFPEA)

Association of Fishers and Lake Users of Uganda (AFALU)

BACKGROUND, AIM AND SUMMARY OF PREVENTATIVE CARE INTERNATIONAL (NGO)

Preventative care international (PCI) is NGO (Non-governmental Organisation) founded in 2013. Aimed at preventing HIV in women, children and adult men.

The PCI Organisation aimed at:

- Aimed at preventing HIV in women, children and adult men
- To have a free community that is free from HIV/AIDS and reproductive health challenges
- We sensitise both rural and urban areas on dangers of STIs, HIV and AIDS

Background

There is no known cure for HIV or AIDS (globally), only treatment to delay HIV from progressing into AIDS. The only way to know whether one has HIV or not is by taking an HIV test. Taking an HIV test helps in making decisions to protect oneself in future. USAID, through PEPFAR, is working to achieve the Joint United Nations Programme on HIV/AIDS' ambitious 90–90–90 global goals by 2020. USAID's HIV and AIDS program has been on the forefront of the global AIDS crisis for 30 years.

Today, more than 36.7 million people are living with HIV worldwide. USAID is a key implementing partner under the U.S. President's Emergency Plan for AIDS Relief (PEPFAR), the largest and most diverse HIV and AIDS prevention, care and treatment initiative in the world. The Office of HIV/AIDS provides global leadership to maximize the impact of USAID's overall response to HIV and AIDS. USAID also supports country-led efforts to combat the complex challenges of HIV and AIDS in 35 countries around the world. By using the Agency's unique health and development perspective, while leveraging our technical expertise, we partner with countries to ensure cost-effective, sustainable, and integrated HIV and AIDS programming that harnesses the latest science and technological innovations all in order to achieve the goal of a world where HIV and AIDS are no longer burdens on health and development.

According to As a result of PEPFAR, USAID and other implementing partners have: Supported lifesaving antiretroviral treatment for more than 14.6 million people. Supported HIV testing for more than 95 million people. Provided care and support for nearly 6.8 million orphans and vulnerable children and their families. Supported training for more than 270,000 healthcare workers to deliver HIV and other health services.

The HIV (Human Immune virus) and AIDS (Acquired Immune deficiency Syndrome) epidemic in Uganda has continued to be a serious public health issue contributing to the high morbidity and mortality rates one the highest incidence and prevalent rates of approximately 1.4 million people with AIDS victims of adults and children in 2018. AIDS has made several people susceptible to infections and diseases for example tuberculosis and cancers due low CD4 counts. In fact out of the 1.4 million people living with HIV, only 900,000 individuals are currently receiving anti-retroviral therapy. Therefore 300,000 individuals of known HIV positive status are in urgent need of starting treatment. This is negatively affecting the country's progress towards attaining the second "90"UNAIDS target.

Uganda registered 83,000 new infections by the end of 2018. This translates to 227 new infections per day. The situation is grave among young people and particularly among young women and girls with the country registering 50 new infections a day in this group or 2 infections per hour. UNAIDS also reported that 570 adolescents and young girls aged 14 to 25 years were getting infected with HIV per week in Uganda[4]. In all age groups, it's evident that young women and girls are more infected/affected by HIV. Furthermore, one in four adolescent girls has either had a child or is pregnant and 58% of adolescent girls have reported physical or sexual violence[6] Currently the HIV prevalence in the general population is estimated at 6% with about 1.5 million living with HIV infection.

At the end of 2018, 3100 children, acquired HIV from their mothers. Today, 9 in 10 HIV positive women who require treatment are receiving it and new infections in children have dropped drastically from 10,000 a year to 3100 by the end of 2018. The science for preventing HIV in babies is well advanced and prevention of mother-to child infection programming is known to be the most cost effective programs which is achievable with limited resources. There is need to consolidate PMTCT /eMTCT progress to ensure that no child is born with HIV in Uganda. We need to ensure that every pregnant woman attends antenatal care in the early stages of pregnancy, delivers from a designated healthcare facility, that HIV positive mothers continue to consistently take their ARVs after they have given birth and that Children are brought back to a healthcare facility to verify their HIV status. Data from UPHIA (Uganda Population HIV Impact Assessments) 2018 identified existing gaps in HIV programs and specific populations that need special focus. HIV prevalence among those aged 15–19 years was 1.1% (1.8% in girls and 0.5% in boys), this increases to 3.3% among those aged 20–24 years (5.1% in young women and, l.3% in young men). It then increases again to 6.3% among those aged 25–29 (8.5% in women and.3.5% in men). This shows that new infections remain an issue in these age groups in current twenty first century challenges. This continuing infection risk necessitates innovative interventions to prevent new infections in young people.

Though adult HIV prevalence among men is estimated at 4.3% compared to women 7.5% (UPHIA 2018), men continue to be drivers of HIV in the community and more so uneducated men. The men's poor health-seeking behaviour results in low uptake of testing, prevention and treatment services among them. Fewer men know their HIV status and those who are HIV positive are not receiving HIV treatment due to negative cultural and behavioral masculinity which encourages multiple and concurrent as well as cross generational sex. This means that there is a group of the population with high HIV viral loads in their bodies living with the virus, serving as channels of unchecked and continued new HIV infections in the general population due to unawareness campaigns and programmes contributing health promotion.

For example in Uganda, a lot of young women and girls involved in sex trade at the main land relocate to fishing communities once there are good fish catches and fisher men are getting more money. With the belief by many fisher men that they can die in the lake any time, they spend their free time merry making and engaging in sex with new young women/girls that come to the landing sites. All this is dome with little and sometimes no knowledge about HIV prevention. Even those who have knowledge about HIV prevention have little or no access to prevention options like condoms, STI (Sexually Transmitted Infection) treatment and HIV treatments.

Many young women and girls are in high risk relationships like HIV serodiscordant relationships but they don't know because their male partners are not willing to go for HIV testing. These young women do not have information and options for HIV prevention. This is not only risky to them and their partners but also to their unborn and breast feeding babies.

HIV prevention

- HIV combined prevention strategy
- Sexual prevention
- Prevention through Blood
- Voluntary medical male circumcision

- Prevention of mother to child transmission
- Post exposure prophylaxis (PEP)
- Pre Exposure Prophylaxis (PrEP)
- ART
- STI treatment

THE COMPREHENSIVE PREVENTION PACKAGE IN UGANDA

HIV combined prevention strategy

- Behavioural: (Behaviour related issues) multiple sexual partners, Alcohol and substance abuse, peer pressure, community perception
- Biomedical: (Medical rerated issues) PMTCT, VMMC, Condom use, ARVs, PEP, PrEP
- Structural: These are Social, cultural, economic, political and environmental issues

Prevention through sex in Uganda

- Know your HIV sero-status
- Reduce on risky habits such as alcohol consumption
- Abstinence: Delay sex until marriage
- Being faithful to one tested HIV negative partner
- Condoms: Correct and consistence
- Disclosure
- Early diagnosis and management of STDs

Benefits of using a condom

- Reduce unwanted pregnancy in addition to HIV
- Prevents HIV and other STDS
- Condoms do not affect future fertility
- Condoms can be used without seeing a health worker

Voluntary medical male circumcision (SMC)

- VMMC is the removal of the skin that covers the head of the penis in a health facility by a trained Medical person
- VMMC creates a thicker and more HIV/STI resistance membrane where the foreskin was
- VMMC does not give full protection against HIV
- ABC should still be practiced
- HIV circumcised men can still transmit HIV
- VMMC should always be conducted in a hygienic environment
- It is dangerous to resume sex before the wound has healed completely after circumcision
- It is important to discuss with your sexual partner

Other health benefits

- Hygiene
- Protection of women against cervical cancer
- Protection of women against STIs

Prevention of mother to child transmission of HIV (PMTCT)

PMTCT is a comprehensive approach that includes:

- HIV counseling and testing: Primary prevention
- Antenatal care
- Condom use
- Provision of ARVs for viral load suppression
- Delivery at the health clinics, hospitals, health centres
- Infant feeding and
- Family planning counseling

Prevention through blood

- Avoid conditions for blood transfusion
- Use screened blood
- Avoid sharing unsterilised sharp skin piercing objects
- Wear protective gears to avoid direct contact with blood

Pre exposure prophylaxis (PrEP)

- PrEP is the use of ARVs by people who are not infected by HIV to prevent HIV infection
- Someone who is not infected with HIV takes a daily pill for prevention before they are exposed to HIV
- PrEP is available in Uganda for people at high risk of infection but in very few sites and we need to scale it up

Post exposure prophylaxis

- Use of medicines against HIV after accidental exposure e.g. Rape, Accidental Needle prick

Procedure

- Done within 72 hours
- HIV counseling and testing
- Negative source and Negative Victim: No
- Negative source and Positive Victim: No
- Positive source and Positive Victim: No
- Positive source and Negative Victim: Yes

Anti-retroviral therapy

- Drugs are used to slow down the replication of HIV
- When used in combination, ARVs delay HIV replication and the deterioration of the immune system thus improving survival and quality

Before starting treatment

When an individual tests positive or diagnosed with HIV, he or she must have regular blood tests to monitor the progress of the HIV infection before starting treatment.

Two important blood tests are:

- HIV viral load test – a blood test that monitors the amount of HIV virus in one's blood
- CD4 lymphocyte cell count – which measures how the HIV has affected in one's immune system

Treatment can be started at any point following an individual's diagnosis or depending on his or her circumstances and in consultation with HIV doctor.

IMPORTANT ASPECTS OF CD4 CELL COUNTS

CD4 cells are white blood cells that play an important role in the immune system. An individual CD4 cell count gives one an indication of the health of his or her immune system.

The human body's natural defence system against pathogens, infections and illnesses.

CD4 cells are sometimes also called T-cells, T-lymphocytes, or helper cells.

An individual CD4 cell count is the number of blood cells in a cubic millimetre of blood (a very small blood sample). It is not a count of all the CD4 cells in a human body. A higher number indicates a stronger immune system.

- The CD4 cell count of a person who does not have HIV can be anything between 500 and 1500.
- People living with HIV who have a CD4 count over 500 are usually in pretty good health.
- People living with HIV who have a CD4 cell count below 200 are at high risk of developing serious illnesses. HIV treatment is recommended for all people living with HIV. It is especially important for people with low CD4 counts.

If an individual has HIV and do not take HIV treatment, his or her CD4 count will fall over time. The lower the CD4 cell count, the greater the damage to the immune system and the greater the risk of illness. When he or she takes HIV treatment, his or her CD4 count should gradually increase.

HAVING YOUR CD4 CELL COUNT MONITORED BEFORE TAKING HIV TREATMENT

- In the past, CD4 cell counts were used to guide decisions about when to start HIV treatment. However, we now know that all people living with HIV can benefit from HIV treatment and that it is better to start treatment sooner, rather than later.
- "When an individual is taking HIV treatment, his or her viral load is a more important indicator of one's health and of the effectiveness of your treatment than your CD4 cell count."

- Monitoring of your CD4 cell count is still important soon after diagnosis with HIV, before beginning HIV treatment and for as long as one's CD4 count is low. It provides important information about disease progression and the immune system.
- If one has chosen not to start HIV treatment for the moment, then keeping an eye on CD4 count will help him or her and one's doctor assess how safe it is to continue without treatment.

For example, if someone's CD4 cell count is 200 or below, he or she are at risk of developing some serious illnesses and infections. One's doctor should recommend that he or she started HIV treatment urgently, without delay.

If he or she has CD4 cell low count, his or her doctor should also offer additional drugs to try prevent these infections, known as prophylaxis. Thus one should take prophylaxis whether or not you take HIV treatment. For example, he or she may need cotrimoxazole (Septrin) to prevent PCP pneumonia until his or her CD4 cell count rises above 200 while on HIV treatment.

If his or her CD4 cell count is low, then one may have some additional tests, for example screening for tuberculosis (TB).

YOUR CD4 CELL COUNT WHEN YOU ARE TAKING TREATMENT

- Once one has started taking HIV treatment, and his or her viral load starts to fall, your CD4 cell count is likely to increase gradually. The rate at which this happens can vary a lot between individuals.
- During one's first months taking HIV treatment, his or her CD4 count will continue to be monitored regularly. Nonetheless when one is taking HIV treatment, one's viral load is a more important indicator of your health and of the effectiveness of his or her treatment than his or her CD4 cell count. After a while, one's doctor may suggest checking his or her CD4 cell count less often.
- If one has had an undetectable viral load for at least a year and his or her CD4 cell count is over 200, then his or her doctor may suggest monitoring their CD4 cell count once a year.
- If one has had an undetectable viral load and a CD4 cell count over 350 for at least a year, then one's doctor may feel that CD4 cell counts are not needed at all; so long as one's viral load remains undetectable.
- However, if one's viral load increased, or has had HIV-related symptoms, then his or her CD4 cell count would be monitored again.

VARIATIONS IN CD4 CELL COUNTS

CD4 cell counts can vary a lot between people. Your own CD4 cell count may go up and down in response to different factors such as exercise, lack of sleep or smoking. But these factors don't seem to make any difference to how well your immune system can fight infections.

Rather than attach too much significance to an individual test result, it makes good sense to monitor any trends in changes to your CD4 cell count over time. It's best to have your CD4 count measured at the same clinic and at roughly the same time of day wherever possible. If you have another infection, such as the flu or an outbreak of herpes, talk to your clinic about whether it is best to delay your CD4 count until you are feeling better. If you get a result that is very different to that expected, your doctor may want to repeat the test to check whether the first result was a laboratory error.

CD4 PERCENTAGE

In addition to using a test to count the number of CD4 cells, doctors sometimes measure the proportion of all white blood cells that are CD4 cells. This is called a CD4 cell percentage. Although it's not recommended that CD4 percentages are used as a general indicator of the health of an adult's immune system, there can be situations where it is a useful measurement. For example, if your CD4 percentage is very different to your CD4 cell count, it might be a sign of another health problem. One circumstance when your doctor might measure your CD4 cell percentage could be if there is a big variation in your CD4 cell count between one test and the next.

TREATMENT AND DRUGS

Antiretroviral (ART) drugs inhibit the growth and replication of HIV. Most treatments for HIV/AIDS are given as several medications in combination. ART regimens typically consist of two nucleoside reverse transcriptase inhibitors (NRTIs) plus a third agent, such as a protease inhibitor (PI), an integrase strand transfer inhibitor (INSTI), or a non-nucleoside reverse transcriptase inhibitor (NNRTI). Plus, a boosting agent may be given to increase the blood levels of certain drugs.

The following tables list the main classes and groups of FDA-approved medications used to treat HIV in the U.S., with a brief description. Drugs and combinations are identified by generic and brand names, as well as common abbreviations. Follow the links to access the most up-to-date Drugs.com drug information such as dosing, side effects, drug interactions and pill pictures for each agent and drug class.

Antiretroviral (HIV) drug therapy list

Antiviral boosters

Generic Name	Brand Name	Abbreviation
ritonavir	**Norvir**	RTV
cobicistat	**Tybost**	COBI

- Antiviral boosters are medicines often used in conjunction with other specific antiviral drugs to enhance or increase their effect
- They might be used in conjunction with the protease inhibitors like darunavir or atazanavir
- Antiviral boosters ensure the correct levels of drug are in the blood

Antiviral combinations

Table 1

Generic Name	Brand Name	Abbreviation
abacavir, dolutegravir, and lamivudine	**Triumeq**	ABC/DTG/3TC
abacavir and lamivudine	**Epzicom**	ABC/3TC
abacavir/lamivudine/zidovudine	**Trizivir**	ABC/3TC/ZDV
atazanavir and cobicistat	**Evotaz**	ATV/COBI
cobicistat and darunavir	**Prezcobix**	COBI/DRV

(Continued)

Generic Name	Brand Name	Abbreviation
cobicistat, elvitegravir, emtricitabine, and tenofovir alafenamide	**Genvoya**	COBI/EVG/FTC/TAF
cobicistat, elvitegravir, emtricitabine and tenofovir disoproxil fumarate	**Stribild**	COBI/EVG/FTC/TDF
efavirenz, emtricitabine, and tenofovir disoproxil fumarate	**Atripla**	EFV/FTC/TDF
emtricitabine, lopinavir, ritonavir, and tenofovir disoproxil fumarate	**AccessPak for HIV PEP Expanded with Kaletra**	FTC/LPV/RTV/TDF
emtricitabine, nelfinavir, and tenofovir disoproxil fumarate	**AccessPak for HIV PEP Expanded with Viracept**	FTC/NFV/TDF
emtricitabine, rilpivirine, and tenofovir alafenamide	**Odefsey**	FTC/RPV/TAF
emtricitabine, rilpivirine, and tenofovir disoproxil fumarate	**Complera**	FTC/RPV/TDF
emtricitabine and tenofovir alafenamide	**Descovy**	FTC/TAF
emtricitabine and tenofovir disoproxil fumarate	**Truvada, AccessPak for HIV PEP Basic**	FTC/TDF
lamivudine and zidovudine	**Combivir**	3TC/ZDV

Main points to remember

- CD4 cell counts give an indication of the health of an individual immune system.
- An individual CD4 cell count should go up when one takes HIV treatment.
- Monitoring CD4 cell counts is less important while taking HIV treatment than before starting.
- No more taking handful of pills multiple times each day. Combinations of HIV treatments – many recently approved – have become more effective, easier to take, and with fewer side effects.
- A person's initial HIV regimen generally includes three HIV medicines from at least two different drug classes. This generally includes two nucleoside reverse transcriptase inhibitors (NRTIs) plus a third agent (PI, INSTI, or NNRTI), and possibly a boosting agent.
- Combination agents can make treatments easier and help patients to take their medication each day as prescribed and adhere to their regimen long term.

Integrase Strand Transfer Inhibitors (INSTI)

Generic Name	Brand Name	Abbreviation
• dolutegravir	• Tivicay	• DTG
• elvitegravir	• Vitekta	• EVG
• raltegravir	• Isentress	• RAL

- Integrase is an enzyme needed by the HIV virus so that it can make copies of itself. Integrase strand transfer inhibitors, also just known as integrase inhibitors, block the action of integrase.
- Integrase strand transfer inhibitors prevent human immunodeficiency virus from multiplying in the host.

Generic Name	Brand Name	Abbreviation
maraviroc	**Selzentry**	MVC

- Chemokine receptor antagonists block the entry of HIV into the host cell, thereby slowing the replication of the virus.

Generic Name	Brand Name	Abbreviation
enfuvirtide	**Fuzeon**	T-20

- Fusion inhibitors like enfuvirtide block HIV's ability to infect healthy CD4 cells.
- When used with other anti-HIV medicines, these drugs can reduce the amount of HIV in the blood, increase the number of CD4 cells, and keep help the immune system healthy so it can fight infection.

Non-Nucleoside Reverse Transcriptase Inhibitors (NNRTIs)

Generic Name	Brand Name	Abbreviation
delavirdine	**Rescriptor**	DLV
efavirenz	**Sustiva**	EFV
etravirine	**Intelence**	ETR
nevirapine	**Viramune, Viramune XR**	NVP
rilpivirine	**Edurant**	RPV

- Non-nucleoside reverse transcriptase inhibitors (NNRTIs), or non-nucleoside analogs, bind directly to reverse transcriptase to prevent conversion of RNA to DNA to keep HIV out of the healthy human cell, and blocks replication.

Nucleoside, Nucleotide Reverse Transcriptase Inhibitors (NRTIs)

Generic Name	Brand Name	Abbreviation
abacavir	**Ziagen**	ABC
didanosine	**Videx, Videx EC**	DDI
emtricitabine	**Emtriva**	FTC
lamivudine	**Epivir**	3TC
stavudine	**Zerit**	d4T
tenofovir disoproxil fumarate	**Viread**	TDF
zidovudine	**Retrovir**	AZT, ZDF

- Nucleoside reverse transcriptase inhibitors (NRTIs), sometimes referred to as nucleoside analogs, were the first antiretroviral drugs to be developed, starting with zidovudine.
- Viread (tenofovir disoproxil fumarate) was the first nucleotide analog reverse transcriptase inhibitor (NRTI) approved for HIV treatment. Both classes work by blocking the reverse transcriptase enzyme crucial to the production and replication of HIV.
- Nucleotide analogs are different from the nucleoside analogs, although they act in much the same way. In order for nucleoside analogs to work, they must undergo chemical changes (phosphorylation) to become active in the body. Nucleotide analogs, like tenofovir, bypass this step because they are already chemically activated.

Protease Inhibitors (PIs)

Generic Name	Brand Name	Abbreviation
atazanavir	**Reyataz**	ATV
darunavir	**Prezista**	DRV
fosamprenavir	**Lexiva**	FPV
indinavir	**Crixivan**	IDV
lopinavir and ritonavir	**Kaletra**	LPV/RTV
nelfinavir	**Viracept**	NFV
ritonavir	**Norvir**	RTV
saquinavir	**Invirase**	SQV
tipranavir	**Aptivus**	TPV

- Protease Inhibitors (PIs) work by interfering with the enzyme HIV protease, which in turn interrupts HIV replication at a later stage in its life cycle. This causes HIV particles in the body to become structurally disorganized and non-infectious.
- PIs can cause a significant number of side effects due to drug interactions with some other medications metabolized by a particular enzyme system in the liver.

Treatment for Pre-Exposure Prophylaxis (PrEP)

Generic Name	Brand Name	Abbreviation
emtricitabine and tenofovir disoproxil fumarate	**Truvada, AccessPak for HIV PEP Basic**	FTC/TDF

- Pre-exposure prophylaxis (PrEP) with antiretroviral medications is a standard treatment that can be used to help prevent new infections among those at high risk for contracting HIV.
- HIV treatment guidelines recommend that PrEP be used for people who are HIV-negative and at substantial risk for HIV infection, including high risk men who have sex with men; high risk transgender women, high risk heterosexual men and women; and high risk injection drug users.
- PrEP, if used correctly, can reduce the risk of HIV transmission by over 90 percent. However, PrEP should be used with counseling on other risk reduction practices, such as correct condom use and safe needle practices.
- Truvada is still the only FDA-approved pre-exposure prophylaxis (PrEP) regimen. In April, 2016, the FDA approved Gilead's Descovy (emtricitabine + tenofovir alafenamide [TAF]), an HIV nucleoside reverse transcriptase inhibitor (NRTI) for the treatment of HIV-1 infection. But unlike Truvada, Descovy is NOT approved for PrEP; it is not yet clear whether Descovy will work as well as Truvada for PrEP. Descovy contains tenofovir alafenamide (TAF) instead of tenofovir disoproxil fumarate (TDF). Phase 3 clinical trials comparing the effectiveness of Truvada to Descovy for PrEP are currently ongoing at prevent.

Art goals

To prolong the survival of PHA, reduce their morbidity and improve quality of life by:

- Suppressing HIV replication/multiplication to as low as possible
- Enhance immune function (CD4 restoration)

Who should take ARVs

- Clinical AIDS regardless of CD4 count
- HIV infected Pregnant mothers

Side effects

- Skin rash
- Dizziness
- Headache
- Nightmares
- Yellow eyes
- Anemia

Summary points of ARVs

- ARVs are life saving
- ARVs make you well again, but do not cure
- ARVs must be taken for life
- Take tablets at the right time
- ARVs may cause unwanted side effects
- Do no stop ARVs unless told to do so
- Disclose to at least a family member
- Agree on treatment supporter
- No skipping or missing tablets

Family planning

- An effort by couples or an individual to regulate number of children and spacing of birth by using family planning methods of their choice

Methods

- Short acting: Condoms, pills, injectables, lactation amenorrhea
- Long acting; Intra uterine device, in plants
- Permanent methods: Tube ligation (Female), Vasectomy (male)

Funding

- Funding from international NGOs is to ensure we continue maintain the PCI and provide services to women and children
- To help support men who also contract HIV or AIDS know how well they can live with a virus
- Also to continue raise awareness in prevention of HIV
- Offer counselling to infected individuals

Why extend HIV prevention and care services with our NGO

In spite of the progress that has been made, the burden of HIV infection in the Uganda is still prevalent. There are groups of people that are disproportionately affected and need special attention since they interact with the general population. The HIV prevalence of 14.9–35% among adult men in urban and rural areas compared to the national average of 8% calls for strategic interventions that are appropriate to these communities.

Lack of HIV and AIDS awareness men's poor health-seeking behavior resulting into low uptake of testing, prevention and treatment services. Fewer men know their HIV status and those who are HIV positive are not receiving HIV treatment due to negative cultural and behavioral masculinity which encourages multiple and concurrent as well as cross generational sex. This is worse in fishing communities because men go fishing at night and during day time they feel that they should sale their fish, rest, engage in sex and merry making. This makes it more difficult for them to be reached with healthcare services. We need to put in place an appropriate strategy that can reach these men since they are the drivers of HIV in these communities.

To address the president's initiative of closing the tap on new infections, consolidating the elimination of mother to child transmission of HIV and accelerate the attainment of 90, 90, 90 targets we need to target communities and groups that are facing a greater burden of HIV with high prevalence. We need to extent HIV prevention options that include information on abstinence, condom use, HIV testing and counseling services, screening and treatment of STIs to young women, girls and men in fishing communities. We need to talk about the benefits of PMTCT/eMTCT, adherence to ART/viral load suppression and create appropriate linkages and follow up systems for people to access treatment and prevention services.

Capacity to reach the fisher folks

Uganda Fish Processors and Exporters Association (UFPEA) and Association of Fishers and Lake Users of Uganda (AFALU) the key stakeholder associations in the fish sector have identified Preventive Care International (PCI) which has been working with fishing communities, young women and girls, Key / priority Populations that include fisher folks, sex workers, truck drivers, and HIV Serodiscordant couples since 2013 as a strategic implementation partner. We work with fishing organizations that have membership of over 1,000,000 fisher folks on Lake Victoria, Kyoga and Lake Albert. PCI has been collaborating with the Association of Fishers and Lake Users of Uganda (AFALU) an umbrella organization for fishers and fish input dealers in the country. AFALU is an association working with the Fisheries Protection Unite (FPU) that HE the President appointed to clear fishing illegalities on all the lakes in the country. Uganda Fish Processors and Exporters Association (UFPEA) has collaborative links with Association of Fishers and Lake Users of Uganda (AFALU) who supply fish to the fish processing factories in the country.

PCI has made over 2000 referrals to healthcare facilities that provide prevention/care services and those carrying out HIV research. We have conducted several out reaches at different landing sites to offer free HIV counselling and testing, distribute free condoms and sharing advocacy information on HIV prevention. We have a network for HIV care/prevention providers, civil society organizations in and around fishing communities that we shall continue to work with to reach out to the fishers.

GOAL AND MAIN OBJECTIVE OF HIV CAMPAIGNS

To reduce on new HIV infections among young women /girls and men in fishing communities and contribute towards 90, 90, 90 targets to eliminate HIV by 2030.

Objectives

- To increase knowledge and demand for HIV prevention and care services among young women/ girls and men in fishing communities
- To ease access and improve uptake of HIV prevention and care services among young women/ girls and men in fishing communities
- To create a strong base of peers/champions who can promote HIV prevention/care and healthcare seeking behaviour among fisher folks
- To reduce on new infections and the burden of HIV among young women /girls and men in fishing communities
- To involve and interest men in VCT and ART so as to close the gap on new infections and reduce HIV related death of men and young women and girls

Methodology

The proposed HIV prevention and care services will start within 20 major landing sites targeting young women and girls, men, those who transact different businesses within the fishing community and Healthcare providers. We shall focus on creating awareness by sharing information about HIV prevention through community outreaches, small group discussions and targeted men access points. Fish suppliers to processing factories who own most of the boats and employ majority of the fishers will be sensitized and used as access points to all fishers. We shall work with women who are involved in artisanal fish processing, fish smoking, bar and restaurant business, sex workers, to reach young women and girls who in most cases are employed in these businesses.

Free HIV testing and counselling will be carried out, free condoms and IEC materials will be distributed. Those found to be HIV infected will be linked to centers that provide ART. We shall liaise with healthcare centers that offer ART to facilitate test and treat for those found HIV positive. We shall develop a referral plan detailing contacts of all those found to be HIV infected or need other treatment and details with phone contact for a person at a care facility.

Young women, girls and men will be reached during community outreaches at landing sites, through peer to peer and snowball method. We shall also share information about the comprehensive guidelines for the treatment and prevention of HIV with health care providers within the fishing communities to empower them to respond to questions and demand from the community.

We shall print, distribute and discuss with the community materials on HIV prevention and care approved by Uganda Aids Commission, hold barazas, information dissemination through local radio/ loud speakers in fishing communities. More emphasis and focus will be on reaching men, young women and girls with messages on abstinence, condom use, HIV testing, PMTCT/eMTCT and STIs testing and treatment. This process and all the questions/concerns from different landing sites will be documented to guide us and other people in HIV programing in other areas and populations in the country.

To achieve the above, the following key activities will be undertaken

Key activities

1. Work with fishing associations to identify and train peer leaders to mobilize men, young women and girls to form Peer support Clubs and Groups
2. Work with Uganda Aids Commission to print out IEC materials and develop fisher folks targeted advocacy messages on HIV prevention and care
3. Conduct targeted outreaches for HIV testing and counselling, small group discussions, condom distribution, information sharing and linkage for ongoing care
4. Document and share with stakeholders lessons learnt, best practices and challenges encountered

Expected results

1) Peer support groups/clubs formation
2) A team of trained peer leaders who can champion and promote HIV prevention /care among men, young women and girls in the fishing communities
3) Increased knowledge, uptake and demand for HIV prevention and care services in the fishing communities
4) Easy access to HIV prevention and care services by young women/girls and men in the fishing communities
5) Reduction of new infections among men, young women and girls in the fishing communities
6) More men involvement in the HIV care and prevention services uptake

Activity plan and time line for reaching out to men, girls and young women in fishing communities

Activity	Jan–April	May–Aug	Sept–Dec	Output
Identifying and train peer leaders to mobilize men, young women and girls				
Strategizing meetings with association leaders	To develop an implementation plan by end of Feb			Activity plan that will guide implementation and assign roles to all stakeholders
Identifying peer leaders	Identify peers per landing site by end of Feb			A total of 120 peer leaders to be identified from 20 landing sites, 6 per landing site
Training peer leaders	Train the peers leaders by mid-March			To have a total of 120 peers leaders trained in HIV care and prevention advocacy and community sensitization
Forming peer support groups/ clubs	Form peer group by end of March			40 peer support clubs will be formed for sustainability. 1 for men and 1 for women per landing site

(Continued)

Activity	Jan–April	May–Aug	Sept–Dec	Output
Developing fisher folks targeted advocacy messages on HIV prevention and care				
Reviewing existing advocacy materials	Review existing material and develop more by mid-March			At least 5,000 brochures, posters and fliers with information appropriate for fishing communities to be printed.
Developing more messages targeting men, young women and girls		Start reaching out to men in peer clubs by April		To reach at least 10,000 men, young women and girls with HIV testing and 2,000,000 with HIV prevention messages.
Printing out materials	To have final material printed by end of March			Up to 5000 posters, brochures and fliers will be printed. 250 to be used at each landing site
Conducting targeted outreaches				
Work with peer groups/ clubs to mobilize men		To form 2 peer clubs formed per landing site by Mid-April		To have 40 peer clubs formed. At least 2 per landing site 1, for men and 1 for women for sustainability
Target men dwelling places to talk about HIV prevention			To reach the targeted number by November	To have at least 300 men tested for HIV and reach 5,000 with HIV prevention messages per landing site
HIV testing and counselling, condom distribution			To have the targeted number of people tested by November	To test and counsel at least 10,000 people and distribute condoms
Linkage to care organizations for ongoing support			To have all the HIV positive people linked to care by mid-December	All those that test HIV positive will be linked to care centers
Sharing lessons learnt, best practices and challenges				
Compiling a report			To have a report by mid-December	One report highlighting best practices, challenges and recommendations shared with UAC, MHO, civil society, researcher s, program implementers and other key stakeholders
Stakeholders meeting to share lessonss/ challenges			To have a stakeholders meeting by December 30	Feedback and recommendation for better service delivery

Targeted landing sites to operate in for the first year			
Region	**Name**	**Population 7/1/2017 Est.**	**Busiest Landing Sites**
Central	Buikwe	445,300	Kiyindi
	Buvuma	106,700	Kirongo
	Kalangala	60,000	Kachanga and Misonzi
	Kalungu	187,700	Kamuwongo
	Kampala	1,583,000	Ggaba
	Masaka	314,000	Lambu, Dimu
	Mpigi	266,400	Kaggulube
	Mukono	643,100	Katosi, Koome Island
	Rakai	252,600	Kasensero and Sango Bay
	Wakiso	2,391,500	Kasenyi and Kigungu
Eastern	Bugiri	426,000	Gorofa and Wakawaka
	Jinja	490,100	Masese
	Mayuge	513,900	Bwondha
	Namayingo	224,800	Mutumba
Total		**7,905,100**	

ACKNOWLEDGEMENTS

I want to acknowledge Charles Brown (Executive Director and Komwiswa Rogers Programs Director) of Preventive International Care. All these played scientific research part and are work colleagues of Preventive International Care (NGO). I want to dedicate this research mainly to those who are victims of HIV and AIDS.

ABOUT THE AUTHORS

Mr. Johnson Mbabazi is a public health specialist, Fellow of the Royal Society of Public Health, Associate of the Royal College of Physicians of Public Health and The European Public Health Association as well as a multi-international award winning author and Plaque winner in UK.

Dr Mohammed Sattar, General Practitioner Partner - Male, MBChB (Sheffield) 2010, MRCGP 2016 at Woodhouse Medical Practice in Leeds, and medical physician at the NHS as well as an author.